In Search of My Father

Dementia is no match for a daughter's determination

Dr Helena Popovic MBBS

Published by Choose Health, Australasia

First published in Australia in 2011
Reprinted in Australia and New Zealand in 2012, 2013, 2014, 2015, 2018, 2020 and 2022

Liability Disclaimer
The material contained in this book is general in nature and does not represent medical advice. It is not intended to provide specific guidance for particular circumstances and it should not be relied on as a basis for any decisions to take action on any matter which it covers. Readers should obtain professional advice before acting on any information in this book. The author disclaims all responsibility and liability to any person, arising directly or indirectly, from any person taking or not taking action based upon the information in this publication.

National Library of Australia Cataloguing-in-publication data:

Author: Popovic, Helena
Title: In Search of My Father: Dementia is no match for a daughter's determination / Helena Popovic
ISBN: 9780994335722 (pbk.)
ISBN: 9780994335715 (ebook)
Notes: Includes bibliographical references.
Subjects: Dementia—Patients—Care. Fathers and daughters.
Dewey Number: 362.19683

Editor: Mark Stafford
Proofreaders: Jean Cooney and Jean Kirkness
Cover Design: Dada Marketing

Dedication

To all my teachers at Meriden School—I can't thank you enough for feeding, stimulating, challenging and rewarding my brain for 13 wonderful years, and for knowing that love comes above. Before this research was even available, you were already applying it.

At the Top

by Michael Leunig

At the top of the tallest building in the world
Sat the saddest man in the world
And inside the man
Was the loneliest heart in the world
And inside the heart
Was the deepest pit in the world
And at the bottom of the pit
Was the blackest mud in the world
And in the mud lay the lightest, loveliest, tenderest,
Most beautiful, happy angel in the universe.

Reproduced with permission from Penguin Books Australia.

About the Author

Dr Helena Popovic MBBS is a medical doctor, award-winning author and international speaker. She is a leading authority on improving brain function, preventing dementia and shedding excess body fat. These subjects are not as disparate as they seem. Midlife obesity and type 2 diabetes double the risk of dementia and avoiding these two conditions will go a long way to averting a dementia epidemic.

Dr Helena graduated from the University of Sydney and her passion is empowering people to live longer, stronger, healthier and happier. Her driving philosophy is that **education is more powerful than medication** and she believes that **our decisions are more powerful than our DNA**. Helena shared her mother's journey with lung cancer and her father's adventure with dementia. She writes and speaks from a personal and professional perspective.

Helena regularly advises Alzheimer's organisations, speaks at Aged Care conferences and trains health professionals in the treatment of dementia. She is a frequent guest on Australian TV, notably Channel 7's *Daily Edition* and Channel 9's *Morning Show* and *Today Extra*.

In 2012 Helena and her father appeared on Channel 7's *Weekend Sunrise* for Dementia Awareness Week. In 2013 Helena was a guest at Auckland Writers and Readers Festival where she spoke alongside Kate De Goldi, and in 2014 she was the key presenter for New Zealand Brain Awareness Week.

In 2017 Helena joined *Talking Lifestyle* Radio 2UE Sydney and 3AW Melbourne for 12 months to create a weekly podcast on how to take control of our health. In 2020 she presented Health-e-Bytes on ABC Radio Gold Coast. You can listen to the recordings at: **www.adventurepreventsdementia.com**

Helena is also unique in bringing the latest discoveries in brain science to weight management. Her groundbreaking program is called *NeuroSlimming—Let your brain change your body*. For more information about how to shed excess body fat without dieting or deprivation, visit: **www.winningatslimming.com**

Contents

Acknowledgements

Every day my Gratitude Journal is filled with thanks and appreciation for the incredibly wonderful people in my life. My friends are my lifeline, my inspiration and my joy. You are too many to name individually, but you are all a gift and a constant source of support and encouragement.

Specifically in relation to this book, I'd like to thank my patient, insightful and meticulous editor, Mark Stafford, who has been an absolute pleasure to work with. Thank you to Jillian Kingsford Smith, social media guru, whose enthusiasm, expertise and optimism sustained my excitement even when I wasn't sure where I was going. Thank you to Matt Church for his capacity to see a person's light even when it only feels like a flicker. Thank you to Craig Bulmer for his tenacity and skill in bringing out the best in people. Thank you to Dale Beaumont, publishing wizard and remarkable entrepreneur, for his comprehensive guidance in getting a book from headspace to shelf-space. Thank you to John Anderson for his fortitude and understanding whenever I changed my mind about what I wanted to convey. Thank you to James Adonis, Kirsty Spraggon, Graeme Cowan and Michelle Bowden, who generously shared their own publishing journeys to pave an easier path for me. Thank you to Rob and Tracey Clarke, founders of LearnX and *Training Australia* magazine for their belief in me and for offering me opportunities for authorship while I was still in the early stages of my research.

An enormous thank you to Associate Professor Peter Thursby for his tireless help with all things computers and Internet—without you I'd still be in the technological dark ages. And thanks to both you and Pat for all your assistance with Dad. Thank you to Dr Andrew Czyniewski for always being there to help with Dad's medical needs, and to Sheila for her selfless, practical aid whenever I need a last-minute chauffeur, minder or pot of soup.

Thank you to Dr Brent Thomas for always managing to put a smile on Dad's face.

Thank you to Joan and Peter, Zoran and Diana for your generosity and hospitality, and for looking after Dad while I cloistered myself in your guest rooms to write for hours on end.

Thank you to Cheryl Rowley for her astute and honest feedback. Your observations provided the basis for a profound turning point in my relationship with Dad—and with myself. It amazes me how one candid conversation can make such an enormous difference. Thank you to Chris Steele for your sensitivity and extraordinary attention to detail—your comments about the manuscript were invaluable. Thank you to Jean Kirkness for not only picking up the slightest inconsistencies in the text, but for your sagacious and practical remarks on style and structure.

Thank you to all the recipients of my self-therapeutic emails, who encouraged me to turn them into a book, and who continue to provide a listening ear and a balanced perspective throughout my journey—thank you to Andy Steele, Angela Leung, Carolyn Dodds, David and Bernice Bratchford, Dianne Gakas, Dimmy Gerangelos, Etta Melman, Frances Turner, Geoff, Joy and John Sirmai, Gil Lovell, Helen and Keith Hughes, Jasmin Tohadze, Jenny Johnson, Julia Galin, Julie Meakes, Karl Hormes, Lee Tsoukalas, Lionel Fifield, Maja Green, Millie Haw, Monique Aarts, Murray Altham, Robin Jamieson, Sarah Woodbury, Steve Bozajian and Tuncer Cimenbicer for your priceless words of wisdom, advice and confidence.

And thank you, Dad, for showing me the joy of being.

Foreword

People are not inspired to act on reason alone ... In a story you arouse your listener's emotion and energy.
Robert McKee

We are the architects and builders of our own brains.

For millennia, however, we were oblivious to our enormous creative capabilities. We had no idea that our brains were changing in response to our actions and attitudes, every day of our lives. So we unconsciously and randomly shaped our brains and our latter years because we believed we had an immutable brain that was at the mercy of our genes.

Nothing could be further from the truth.

The human brain is continually altering its structure, cell number, circuitry and chemistry as a direct result of everything we do, experience, think and believe. This is called "neuro-plasticity".

With a wealth of research and clinical experience as its foundation, this book began as a step-by-step guide to moulding our brains into life-long, peak performers. A peak performing brain means we're sharp, focused, creative and resilient. It means we're fast learners, resourceful thinkers and effective problem solvers. It means we have a good memory for the duration of our lives. It means we substantially reduce our risk of degenerative brain disorders, such as Alzheimer's Disease, other dementias, stroke and depression. It means we remain in possession of our mental faculties and live meaningful, fulfilling lives until our last days. And the best news of all is that we're never too old, too young or "too far gone" to make positive, life-expanding, extraordinary changes.

This book isn't just about preserving brain function as we age—it's about enhancing performance, effectiveness, health and joy at every age and stage of life.

However, the book took a different direction when my mother died and I was left to care for my frail, elderly father in the early stages of dementia. Full of energy, enthusiasm and scientific arrogance, I set about to redesign my father's brain. But life has a way of interfering with our plans. I found I was not dealing with a willing, motivated patient, but a grief-stricken, self-doubting man. And I underestimated the impact of the experience on my own life. Eventually I stopped resisting the hand that life had dealt me, and learned to fuse my personal trials with my medical training.

The result is this book, which weaves science into story, reflection into research, past into present and humour into healing. The interplay of science and personal story (in which the names have been altered to respect privacy) allows you to switch from analytical, left brain evaluation of the facts to a right brain, creative exploration of the possibilities for your own life. Stories are more powerful in effecting change and making messages stick than is straight knowledge. Knowing something is great; implementing knowledge is the real goal.

> *If history were taught in the form of stories,*
> *it would never be forgotten.*
> Rudyard Kipling

Part I
Of Mice and Men

The best laid schemes o' Mice an' Men,
Gang aft agley …
(The best laid schemes of Mice and Men oft go awry)

So what?

Adapted from *To a Mouse* by Robert Burns

Intention

If you smile when no-one else is around, you really mean it.
Andy Rooney

It was the week before Christmas 2009. I woke up knowing it was going to be a good day.

A friend had stayed overnight at my place and after she drove off in the morning, I went for a short jog to pick up my car from the nearby, colourful suburb of West End in Brisbane. All the parking in my street is only for two hours, so to prevent my friend from getting a parking fine, I'd moved my car from the garage the previous day so she could park her car there overnight. My car would be safe and sound in a leafy street, 15 minutes' jog away.

When I arrived at my car, I noticed a piece of paper caught under the windscreen wipers, which I duly pocketed to place in the recycling bin when I got home. But as I went to bin it, I saw it was a parking ticket for $50. I looked at the date and noticed it was today's date. How strange. Given that I'd checked very carefully to make sure there were no parking meters and no signs saying I couldn't park in the street, the ticket couldn't be mine. It must have blown off someone else's car some distance away and landed on my windscreen. The only thing contradicting this theory was the fact that my vehicle registration number was printed on the ticket. A quick call to the Council would clear things up immediately, I thought. After all, this was going to be a good day.

I soon discovered that a quick call to the Council is never quick. After wading through various unconcerned automated voices (which nonetheless professed to be concerned) in the Council's phone system, I was finally greeted by the cheerful James. I explained that an error had occurred in the issuing of a parking ticket.

"No, there's been no error," James pointed out, with the same level of concern as the automated voices. "You were in a two-hour parking zone."

"But there were no signs anywhere in the street saying it was a two-hour parking zone." I knew I was right.

"That suburb is classified as a two-hour parking zone unless otherwise stated," said James.

"But how am I supposed to know that?" I protested. "At no time when I sat for my driver's licence was I told I needed mind-reading skills."

"Surely you would have noticed the parking zone signs as you entered the suburb," he suggested.

"Surely if I'd noticed I wouldn't have parked there for more than two hours."

"Then it's unfortunate you didn't notice," James offered.

There was a long pause. I changed tack.

"So is there anything else that has a two-hour time limit in that area? If I go for a swim in the local pool, will I be thrown out after two hours? I don't want to get caught out again."

James ignored my facetiousness and repeated his regret at my failure to notice the parking signs.

"Yes, it's very unfortunate that I didn't notice," I agreed. "I'll never park there again. Given my remorse for breaking a rule of which I was totally unaware, I'd like to have the penalty waived."

"I am in no position to make any decision about your case. If you want to take this further, I suggest you write to the Appeals Review Officer. The address is on the back of the infringement notice."

So I did. As I finished my letter outlining why my penalty should be waived, a rush of goodwill came over me and I added a Merry Christmas wish for all at the Council. Then, as I was putting the letter in an envelope, another rush of something came over me and I took out a Christmas card so that I could write a longer message of warmth to all at the Council. I stapled the letter to the card and ran to the nearest post-box.

As I was walking home, I got the giggles. I imagined what the person opening the card and letter would think and started laughing even more. Passers-by turned to look at me as though I were mad. I laughed even harder at the thought of explaining to them why I was laughing, and by the time I arrived home I'd completely lost it. I can't remember the last time I laughed so much.

I'd set out to dispute a $50 parking fine but I'd also written the letter because I'd decided at the start of the day it was going to be a good day. That meant I was going to be proactive about *making* it good, both consciously and subconsciously. I didn't care about the fine anymore—the laugh was worth it and it was a cheap price to pay to be reminded of the power of intention.

That afternoon, I decided that instead of composing a list of New Year resolutions (which less than 2 per cent of people adhere to anyway), I'd write an intention for 2010:

2010 is a great year, the year when everything falls into place. I'm doing what I love, making a positive difference to my fellow humans and leaving the smallest possible carbon footprint in the process. My new career brings more success and fulfilment than I ever could have imagined, and everything in my world is conspiring to bring me closer to my goals.

I could hardly wait.

Luck

*Maybe I'm lucky to be going so slowly because I might be going
in the wrong direction.*
Ashleigh Brilliant

On the seventh of January every year, I fly to Sydney from
Brisbane—or wherever I happen to be in the world—to celebrate
Serbian Orthodox Christmas at my parents' home. The Serbian
Orthodox Church still uses the Julian calendar, as opposed to
the Gregorian calendar used by the rest of Christendom. Their
respective years are of slightly different lengths, and over
the centuries the Julian calendar has been playing catch-up. I
don't know why the Serbs didn't switch over with the rest of
the Christian world. My father, Ilija, said it was because Serbs
don't waste their time and energy making changes that aren't
necessary. My mother said it was because they were lazy.

Personally, I found the date discrepancy very convenient. As a
child it meant I received two lots of presents because my parents
believed in assimilating into Australian culture, but they were
equally intent on preserving their customs from the fatherland.
As an adult it meant my partner and I could spend "Australian"
Christmas with his family and Serbian Orthodox Christmas with
my family. Everyone was happy.

But this year, on returning home after the obligatory feasting, I
was greeted by a bewildering scene. The electrical safety switch
in my unit had tripped, the fridge had defrosted, the food had
spoiled, the oven was malfunctioning, the toilet was leaking and
a cockatoo had ripped up my Bird of Paradise plant! Fortunately,
this new year was going to be a great year, where everything in
my world conspired to bring me closer to my goals, so I calmly
spent an hour unplugging and systematically re-plugging every
appliance I owned, to find out what had tripped the switch. The

culprit was the dishwasher. I immediately rang the electrician, the dishwasher man, the oven man and the plumber.

The electrician said there was no need for his services; it was a dishwasher problem. The dishwasher man said he would not visit until the electrician had checked that everything was safe. The oven man said he wouldn't work in a kitchen with potentially hazardous electrical circuitry. The plumber turned up because by then I'd learnt not to mention I had any other problems.

The plumber stopped the leak, but after he left I discovered that he'd also stopped the toilet from flushing. I called him back.

"Why didn't you tell me it wasn't flushing when I was there earlier?" he asked.

"Because until you fiddled with it, the toilet *was* flushing."

Another half hour of fiddling and I had a toilet that grunted and groaned but eventually flushed. Meanwhile, I'd convinced the dishwasher man to come the next morning. He took a quick look under the machine and announced, "The capacitor is cracked."

"What does that mean?"

"It's no big deal," he replied. "A capacitor is a waste of time anyway. I'll just create a circuit to bypass it and she'll be sweet."

"If it's redundant, why is it there?"

"It's just to reduce white noise. It stops your TV getting funny lines across it if you have the dishwasher running at the same time. But most TVs are nowhere near the dishwasher, so it isn't necessary."

"Why did it crack?" I asked.

"Dunno. They just do. It happens all the time."

"It sounds like a design fault."

"Well, no, it just happens."

"But things going wrong, which the consumer has to pay to get fixed, shouldn't 'just happen'," I reasoned.

"It's normal for things to wear out and break after a while," dishwasher man said.

"No, it's not normal," I insisted. "If your leg just wore out and broke after a few years of walking, without you falling over or anything, would you consider that normal?"

"No."

"So why should it be normal for a dishwasher part to break down?"

"Dunno. It just does."

In half an hour the job was done and he turned his attention to the oven—fortunately, dishwasher man was also oven man. The problem with the oven was a broken thermostat. Here we go again, I thought.

"Why did it break?"

"Dunno. They just do. It happens all the time."

"It sounds like another design fault."

"Well, no, it just happens."

"But things going wrong, which the consumer then has to pay to get fixed, shouldn't 'just happen'."

"It's normal for things to wear out and break after a while."

We had exactly the same conversation about the thermostat as for the capacitor. Dishwasher/oven man went down to his van to get a replacement thermostat but returned without one. He didn't have the part after all so I would need to book another service call tomorrow. But he did have a bill.

"Here's the call-out charge and labour for the dishwasher, and here's the call-out charge and labour for the oven," he explained.

"Excuse me? Why am I paying a second call-out charge for the oven when you were already here?"

"Because that's the call-out charge."

"But you've already charged me a call-out charge on the dishwasher invoice."

"Yes, and this is the call-out charge for the oven."

It took a while, but I explained that I was not paying two call-out charges, nor a third when the thermostat arrived, whenever that would be. He reluctantly agreed to just one.

But I was still not happy with the toilet. I rang the plumber again.

"Sometimes it's better to just leave things well enough alone," he insisted.

"A constantly leaking toilet is not well enough," I suggested.

He returned and wrestled with the cistern. He emerged from the bathroom dripping with perspiration (or recycled water) and declared it fixed. I did a quick check before he left and, yes, the toilet was flushing. He left an angry plumber.

But it was soon obvious that all was not well in the bathroom. The toilet was now completely dry. This time *I* broke into a cold sweat. But I had to do it—I rang the plumber again.

"I just have a quick question. Could you tell me why the toilet might not be refilling with water?"

"Oh, that just means I didn't flick the valve back," he replied. "All you have to do is unscrew the flush, take the lid off, look for a small plastic lever on the right-hand side near some tubing and flick it the other way. When you screw the flush button back down, make sure you don't do it any tighter than it was when you took it off."

"Um … I'd rather leave that sort of thing to an expert …"

The long-suffering plumber returned, and although we exchanged little more than sideways glances, I soon had a toilet that flushed. Tick. And a toilet that refilled. Another tick. But I also had a toilet that required me to use a screwdriver to wedge the flush button up after flushing, otherwise it flushed indefinitely. I decided to leave well enough alone.

The day surely couldn't get any longer. That evening, I ate dinner, turned on the newly repaired dishwasher, and spent a couple of quiet hours at my desk. When I returned to the kitchen, there was something amiss. It was underwater! It was at times such as this that I was grateful I lived a self-indulgent, child-unencumbered life, so I had the luxury of taking a deep breath, walking outside, looking up at the stars and quoting *Hamlet*: *There is nothing either good or bad, but thinking makes it so.*

Was all this payment for a karmic debt I had accumulated? Or several debts over several lifetimes? In which case, my gratitude should be amplified by the fact that I was wiping the slate clean. No doubt all this was necessary for the new year to be a great year. And there were other reasons to be thankful: the water had not reached the carpet; the electricity was still on; and … that's enough gratitude for one evening.

Let me just clarify that I wasn't *forcing* myself to think *positively*; I was *choosing* to think *constructively*. Long ago I'd come to the conclusion that lucky people were no luckier than unlucky people. It was simply their perception of themselves—lucky people had different conversations with themselves than unlucky people. If a person who labels themselves as lucky stubs a toe, they immediately say to themselves, "Lucky I didn't break my leg." And they feel cheerful. If a person who labels themselves as unlucky stubs a toe, their internal conversation sounds something like, "Why do I always seem to injure myself? It's not fair. That really hurt!" And they feel disgruntled.

Our quality of life is determined by the conversations we have in our heads. At heart, I was a pragmatist and wanted to be happy. So why not play mind games with myself that would lift my spirits, as opposed to dampen them?

My kitchen didn't clean itself. For over an hour, I mopped, washed and dried everything within sight, while chanting a mantra of love and peace to all the tradesmen cradling beers in front of their TVs. By the end of the week, my appliance issues were put to rest. My less enjoyable challenges were out of the way, and I was now ready for the good stuff to come pouring in.

This new year was going to be a great year.

Tunnel Vision

Let us not look back in anger, nor forward in fear,
but around in awareness.
James Thurber

On 7 February 2010, Australians marked the first anniversary of their worst peacetime disaster, the Black Saturday bushfires.

On 7 February 2010, an anti-whaling ship, the *Bob Barker*, collided with a Japanese whaling vessel in the icy waters off Antarctica.

On 7 February 2010, a blizzard battered Washington DC, knocking out power to thousands of homes, and record snowfall was predicted.

On 7 February 2010, Americans reflected on what would have been Ronald Reagan's 99th birthday and how his policies were still affecting their country.

On 7 February 2010, President Obama assured despondent Democrats that he would not abandon his commitment to overhauling health care.

On 7 February 2010, giant feral pigs were discovered polluting the drinking water of Australian cities, sparking a cull.

On 7 February 2010, NSW Government officials and bureaucrats were accused of using $200 million of taxpayers' money to rent some of Sydney's most prestigious offices.

On 7 February 2010, a high-flying Sydney banker was found to have stolen $7 million from his employer, allegedly to spend on prostitutes and gifts for them.

On 7 February 2010, a man accused of stalking actress Keira Knightley was arrested.

On 7 February 2010, two bank robbers masquerading as Muslim women held up a post office near Paris.

On 7 February 2010, the only thing *I* knew was that my mother had died.

Sentence

Every issue, belief, attitude or assumption is precisely what stands between you and your relationship to another human being—and between you and yourself.
Robert Collier

Sixteen months before February 2010, my mother had been diagnosed with lung cancer. It was a chance finding during an ultrasound, which she'd undergone to check for gallstones. The ultrasonographer had inadvertently moved the probe above her diaphragm, where he noticed a suspicious mass. My mother was referred for a biopsy and within a few days had a diagnosis of Stage 3A non-small cell carcinoma with hilar lymph node involvement. As a doctor herself, she knew without asking that the odds of surviving longer than 18 months were less than 25 per cent.

I was at a medical conference when I received the call.

"I have something to tell you but promise me you won't tell your father."

I scowled. I had told my parents years ago I would no longer be the repository of information they wanted to keep from each other. "I don't have time for this right now. I'm in the middle of a conference."

"Yes, you *do* have time for this. I wouldn't be interrupting you if it wasn't important. I have inoperable lung cancer. I'll be starting chemo and radiotherapy next week."

I felt as if I'd been kicked in the stomach. This couldn't be real.

"What? No! When? How?" I choked on the last word.

"I hadn't thought anything of the recurrent bronchitis I'd been getting for six months, but obviously it was a sign that something was wrong."

"Why inoperable? What stage? How far has it spread?" My voice was trembling now.

"Stage 3A, about 10 cm in diameter and confined to my right lobe but it's invaded the lymph nodes."

"So it hasn't spread beyond the lungs?"

"I don't know. I'm getting a full body scan tomorrow."

I swallowed audibly and out of nowhere, scenes from my childhood bombarded me. I felt like a child again, as though my own life was threatened, and a draught coursed through my body. Between us, Mum and I had decades of medical experience to draw on—and yet I felt utterly helpless. The sense of lack of control was very unfamiliar and uncomfortable, and disconcerting territory for both of us.

"I'll fly down tonight."

"No, stay in Brisbane. I'll let you know when I need you. There's no point wasting your time now. There'll be plenty for you to do later."

My family wasn't into being there "just" for support. If there was a job to be done or a duty to be fulfilled, I was expected to be there. Otherwise it was business as usual.

The draught seemed to knot up my internal organs. I wanted to hug my mother, to be hugged, to wind back the clock, to change something—anything—that might have averted this moment.

"And how is Dad not supposed to know all this? You don't think he'll notice your hair falling out?"

"Of course he knows I have a tumour, but he doesn't know it's a death sentence."

"It's not a death sentence! One in four people are alive five years later."

"Three in four people are dead within two years."

Mum's words gutted me. I was terrified she'd already resigned herself to dying. I was desperate for her not to give up. "Since when have you been a conformist? You're always breaking the mould," I reminded her with pride. "When we arrived in Australia, you were told you'd be lucky to get a job washing dishes in a hospital, let alone practising medicine. And what did you reply? 'If I wash dishes for a living, it'll be because I *choose* to and it won't be in a hospital—it'll be in the best restaurant in Sydney!' And within a few years you were *running* a hospital. Three decades later you were receiving an Order of Australia. The odds of that are much lower than one in four."

My panic subsided somewhat. We'd get through this. What had I been thinking? I switched to problem-solving mode: this was an opportunity for healing on many levels and it would bring us closer. Life never gives us more than we can handle.

My mother interrupted my self-soothing. "This is different."

"But if you approach that tumour with the same attitude that you approached your career, it'll be gone before you even start chemotherapy. No-one and nothing messes with you!"

I could hear her trying to smile. "Tell that to your father," she replied. "He needs hope. He'll fall apart otherwise. And don't mention anything to anyone else."

"Why not?"

"I don't want my enemies to celebrate and I don't want my friends to suffer."

"I don't see any of your friends or acquaintances anyway."

"I don't want you telling any of *your* friends either. Word gets around. This is to be kept within the family."

"I'm going to have to tell my work when I start flying down to Sydney for weeks at a time."

"Tell them your father is unwell. They don't have to know the details."

"I don't have that kind of relationship with the people in my life."

"What about the relationship you have with your mother? I would think that comes above any of your other relationships."

Paradigms

You see things; and you say, 'Why?' But I dream things that never were; and I say, 'Why not?'
From *Back to Methuselah* by George Bernard Shaw

So began a year of furtive trips to Sydney to drive my mother to radiotherapy, to keep my father's spirits up during chemotherapy, to attend weddings and other obligatory functions as the family representative, and to prevent people from visiting so they wouldn't discover how sick my mother was. It was part and parcel of being the only child of migrant parents. I think half the people in my life thought I was having an affair and I'm sure Qantas appreciated the extra revenue I contributed.

Even so, my mother was sparing in her requests for my assistance. She told a select few about her illness, so that she'd have a pool of drivers to take her to therapy. Occasionally my father drove her but his skills behind the wheel had deteriorated and she preferred him to stay home. In due course I had to tell my friends and workmates what was going on, swearing them to the same inane secrecy my mother had sworn *me*. The secrecy seemed inane to me, but in my mother's mind it was the best way to handle the situation. Perhaps she felt it was her last vestige of control. Perhaps having people fuss over her would keep reminding her she was unwell. Perhaps she wanted to be remembered as strong and vivacious. Why had I not been more understanding at the time?

During the months that followed Mum's diagnosis, my emotional life went into hibernation. Every time I wanted to cry I felt it was "not a good time", so I swallowed my tears and they eventually dried up. I became numb. Once I became aware of the numbness, it scared me more than having an "inappropriate emotional outburst", but by then it was too late. No feelings were forthcoming. I was a highly functional shell of a person.

Although my mother and I were both medical doctors, we practised under two very different paradigms. My mother took as gospel everything her professors, her science and her biostatistics told her. For her treatment, she wanted the highest dose of the highest potency drugs available; she wanted nothing of support groups, counselling or meditation. As a staunch adherent of mainstream Western medicine, she would fight only with what she regarded as "proven armamentarium".

Her mindset was understandable given that she had no time to waste. And it would have been a great thing if mainstream Western medicine was offering her a cure. But it wasn't. She was acutely aware that she was only buying time, and a limited amount at that. She was angry that the calling she'd dedicated her life to was now failing her. She had given to medicine her heart and soul, her passion and energy, her commitment and loyalty. In her hour of need, it had little to offer her in return.

"Cancer is a shit and my body has betrayed me," my mother declared, looking up at me with tear-soaked eyes. I squeezed her hand.

As for me, I believe Western medicine is excellent at alleviating symptoms and managing emergencies, acute conditions, broken bones and severed parts. It's brilliant at describing the biochemical mechanisms underlying a malfunctioning system. And it's great at keeping us alive long enough to get to the *real* source of an illness—an interplay of familial, cultural, social, environmental, psychological, emotional and behavioural factors. In the words of Edgar Cayce, America's most renowned medical psychic, "spirit first, mind follows, body belongs".

I believe that science is no match for the human spirit. The language of medicine should be one of love, not war. Instead of speaking of *fighting* the infection, *battling* against cancer and *struggling* with weight loss, why not focus on *caring* for our bodies, *listening* to our needs and *feeling* our feelings? (At this time, the irony of my own absent feelings was not lost on me.) In war there are always casualties on both sides, and the same applies when we fight our bodies—even if it's in the name of a cure.

At this point I should explain how I use the term "healing", as opposed to curing. Healing is more than a restoration of physical health. It means recognising ourselves as whole and complete, and accepting and embracing every part of ourselves— unconditionally. Healing means feeling at peace with ourselves and with life. It then becomes the foundation upon which cure of disease is possible.

The body has an intrinsic capacity to repair itself, if we let it. Exactly how we go about "letting it" is the billion dollar question. I believe it's a unique journey for all of us. The journey begins with believing we have answers within us, asking ourselves "What now?" and then keeping still long enough to hear the response. But how to keep still? Does that mean meditating? Taking a walk in the bush? Drawing a picture of nothing in particular? Sitting quietly and listening to the sea? Bringing our awareness to the present moment?

Voltaire observed, "The art of medicine consists of amusing the patient while nature cures the disease." Together with *primum non nocere*—first do no harm—this was the most important advice I was given in my medical training. To realise healing is to awaken a deep respect and awe for the human body and the human experience, so that we're filled with gratitude and inspired to look after ourselves in the best possible way.

Laughter, forgiveness, compassion, empathy and living in the moment are as powerful as chemo and radiotherapy.

Unconditional acceptance of another human being is the most healing thing one person can offer another, yet I struggled to offer it to my mother. In part this was because I felt completely ineffectual and powerless. I wanted to be able to *do* something that would make a difference to her prognosis. I felt that if only I knew the "right" thing to say, it would help her change course. Even though my emotions were buried, they were clouding my perspective. I wanted to be able to listen to her without judgement, without wanting her to do more or be more than she was. But it took me until the eve of her death to finally just *be* there and to recognise that my being there—not doing or saying something—was what she needed.

Kaleidoscope

Confusion is a word we have invented for an order which is not yet understood.
Henry Miller

Denial is an insidious, underhand beast. In spite of the prognosis that hovered over my mother, in spite of the brain metastases, the pleural effusions, the dwindling appetite and the recurrence of lesions in her lymph nodes, I could not—would not and dared not—believe she was dying. My mother, my father and I drifted in and out of denial, as though driving through a fog. Every so often the fog would lift for one of us, prompting one of the other two to grab the steering wheel and head straight back into the thickest cloud.

My mother would not allow the *P* word to be spoken (palliation: treatment to alleviate symptoms or lessen pain, without actually curing the underlying medical condition). Right until her last days, she entreated her oncologist to give her more chemo-therapy, notwithstanding his refusal on the grounds that her body was too weak to cope with it. Dad took the oncologist aside and asked if he'd give her a placebo and just call it chemotherapy, to raise her spirits, to give her hope, to trick her mind into curing her.

My tears could have flooded the ward—but it still wasn't a good time.

We never spoke about what she wanted posthumously. I remember the week after her passing only as dizzying, kaleidoscopic images. The house looked like the perversely colourful remains of a carnival after a bomb blast. Flowers, cards, cakes, tea bags, newspaper clippings, soup bowls, prayer books, Bibles, photos, compression stockings, tissues, handbags, slippers, blankets and more tissues were strewn from one end of the house to the other. Landline stuck to one ear, mobile phone to the other. Typing up the order of service. A nap between 4 am and 5 am. Dozens of devoted friends vying for a part in the gala production. A meal of a handful of spaghetti, forget the fork. *Eight* pall bearers? Any fewer and someone would miss out. Why haven't you chosen clothes for her to wear in the coffin? Yes, accessories as well. A constant barrage of visitors, from morning till morning. A feeling of seasickness. The ghost of a terror-stricken, lost child; hang on, that was my father. My mother had worked in a Catholic hospital for 38 years, so of course it had to be a Catholic service. St Mary's Cathedral isn't available on the date you asked for. Can you scan all the photos? Who's doing the eulogy? Which version of *The Lord is My Shepherd*? I can't get hold of the organist. Do we really need a soloist? Yes, you can compose your own prayers. The first reading is from 1 Corinthians. If you want to view the body, you have to do it *now*. What's an offertory procession? Great, that means I can hand out a few more roles. My father won't have closure unless it's a Serbian Orthodox funeral. Her longest standing friend can propose the toast at the wake. I have no idea how many people will be there. Which menu? That should be enough finger food. No deep-fried foods, please. I don't know whether she wanted a Serbian Orthodox funeral or a Catholic funeral. No, we didn't talk about it. She didn't tell me anything; only that I should wear my slippers when I got up to help her during the night. What do you mean the Serbian Orthodox Church doesn't allow cremation? Dad spoke to his cousin in Belgrade and it's acceptable in Serbia. How can the rules in Australia be more stringent than the rules in the country of origin?

In the end, since I didn't want to get it wrong, we had two funerals and two wakes. The first three Serbian Orthodox priests I contacted regretted they could not perform a funeral service if the body was to be cremated. I told the fourth priest that after the Orthodox funeral, my mother's body would be returned to the funeral parlour to rest over the weekend, before being taken to the Catholic funeral. He didn't ask what would happen after that, so I secured a bearded priest. The only Serbian caterers I found were Croatian, but the food was the same and no-one was the wiser.

On the night after the second funeral, I slept for 14 hours straight.

Denunciation

There is nothing wrong with being afraid, but there is nothing more wrong than allowing that to be your master.
Bobby Darin

Dean was my mother's childhood friend. He was six years older than my mother, and they grew up together in the small vineyard town of Vršac, 85 kilometres northeast of Belgrade. Vršac was a melange of Serbs, Germans and Hungarians, and Dean and my mother lived in the German sector. Dean migrated to the United States and settled in Los Angeles, seven years before my family came to Australia. My parents, my maternal grandmother and I visited Dean in Los Angeles several times, but despite repeated invitations to come and see us in Australia, he never made it until a few days before my mother died.

I drove Dean straight from the airport to the hospital, where my mother was eagerly waiting for him. The delight on her face—and in her whole body—when she saw him made me want to cry. But of course, it wasn't a good time.

If it hadn't been for Dean, I don't know what would have become of my father during the race against time, tradition, technology and physiology that constituted the funeral preparations. I was aware of my father's presence as a hazy, shuffling, disoriented body to which I delegated a few menial tasks, like fixing a door handle that had flown off in the fury. It was Dean who kept him alive when he would have given anything to be dead.

The morning I awoke from my 14-hour hibernation, I stumbled into the kitchen to find Dean imploring my father.

"But you still have a daughter who needs you." Dad just shook his head. He looked like a blanched corpse.

"Of all people," Dean continued, "I know what you're going through. When my first wife died of breast cancer, I couldn't imagine life without her. I remember just focusing on getting through one hour at a time. I never knew one hour could drag on for so long. Life's cruel like that—normally time flies by way too quickly, but when you're in the depths of misery, time slows down to rub in the agony."

My father was in all-consuming pain. The gentle wisps of white hair were a jumbled nest on his head. He'd always been proud of the fact that he'd retained a generous helping of natural hair; he was now clutching handfuls of curls to hold his head off the table. He rocked back and forth in his chair. "I can't face the days and I can't face the nights. Why have I been punished like this?"

"Punishment has nothing to do with it," replied Dean. "There's nothing anyone can say or do to lessen the pain. Time eventually does an about-face and helps you through."

"I can't see why I've been left on this earth. What cruel God wanted to leave me here on my own? I don't want to go on."

"You don't have a choice and you're not on your own. You have your daughter."

"I'm on my own."

I was stunned. Shocked. Disbelieving. Angry and guilt-ridden. I thought my father and I had a good relationship. My mother was the parent I had spent decades trying to understand, appease and get closer to. The relationship with my mother was the one that had consumed most of my emotional and mental energy. How could I have got it so wrong?

Loss

*It's incredibly easy to get caught up in an activity trap, in the
busyness of life, to work harder and harder at climbing the
ladder of success only to discover it's leaning
against the wrong wall.*
Stephen Covey

When I was growing up, Dad and I were the children in
the family; my mother and maternal grandmother were the
disciplinarians. Whenever we drove anywhere, Dad and I would
sit in the back seat of the car, giggling about something my
mother and grandmother were invariably complaining about.
One day we were at the beach and Dad and I had climbed onto
a large, shell-coated rock to look out over the ocean. Suddenly,
a huge wave lunged out of the water, tossed us in the air and
slammed us against the rock. When the foam retreated, I rolled
out of my father's arms, completely unscathed. I turned towards
him and gasped. His athletic body was covered in profusely
bleeding cuts and gashes, imprints of the shells he'd shielded me
from. My mother was furious at both of us.

Dad helped me compose the arguments for my first school
debate. The topic was "TV is bad for us" and I was last speaker
for the affirmative. I closed with an Aesopian fable my father had
told me.

Aesop's master, Xanthus, had invited his disciples to lunch and
he said to Aesop, "You must buy what is good and sweet, the
best that you can find." So Aesop went to the market and bought
hogs' tongues, which he cooked and put on the table.

"What do you mean by bringing us tongue?" asked Xanthus.

Aesop replied, "What is better or sweeter than tongue? A tongue can soothe, heal, educate, advise, praise and express love. There is no greater good than this."

The next day, Xanthus ordered Aesop, "Bring me the worst and most meagre thing you can find. My disciples are to dine with me again."

Again Aesop went to the market and bought hogs' tongues, which he cooked and put on the table.

"What do you mean by bringing us tongue *again*?" asked Xanthus.

"Can you find anything worse or more stinking than tongue?" Aesop replied. "A tongue can offend, lie, damage, torment and destroy love. There is no greater evil than this."

So it is with TV, I argued in the debate. "The opposition maintains that TV is good for us—it *can* be, but that doesn't negate the fact that TV is also bad for us."

We won the debate. How then did I lose my father? I hadn't even known it until I'd lost my mother.

Silence

A subtle thought that is in error may yet give rise to fruitful inquiry that can establish truths of great value.
Isaac Asimov

Dean stayed with us for a week after the funerals, and then we were enveloped by stillness. My father and I were alone—for the first time. It was like stepping out of a crowded disco where the music had been too loud, the lights too garish and the air too stifling. My ears were still buzzing and my head was gyrating. Everyone had tiptoed back to their normal lives—their families, their jobs, their frustrations with mobile phone networks—but for Dad, nothing could ever be normal again.

"I don't want to live without your mother," he declared.

"I know."

"Help me."

"I'll help you—but not like that."

"There's no other way you can help me."

I didn't know what to say. I reached for his hand, but he flinched as though I'd zapped him with electricity. We just sat. After a while I brought a bowl of grapes to the table.

"I don't want to eat anything."

"I know. Just have a little."

"What's the point?"

"You'll feel even worse if you don't eat."

"That's not possible. Besides, I'm holding you up from your life." The tone of the last two words was scathing. "The sooner I'm gone, the better for you."

"You can't really believe that. You talk to me as though you think I don't love you. Do you really think that?"

He sighed heavily, forlornly, the first of many disconsolate sighs. Over the following months, his sighing would drive me to distraction.

"It's not that you intentionally don't love me," he continued. "It's that you're incapable of love. You *think* you know what love is but you have no idea."

"So what *is* love?" I ventured.

He shook his head. "It isn't something you should need to ask. You should just know."

"Well, obviously I *don't* know, so how about you enlighten me?"

"You're frighteningly similar to *my* mother. She wasn't capable of love either." He paused reflectively. "You don't really care about anyone except yourself. You live a very selfish life. No husband, no children, no pets. No concern for your mother and me. You've lived either interstate or overseas for half your life. You just do as you please, when you please and with whom you please. You have no strong connections with anyone. You'll die sad and lonely—like I will."

Now would have been a good time to cry, but of course no tears were there.

Aftershock

What is right is often forgotten by what is convenient.
Bodie Thoene

About a month after the funeral, two Serbian women who my father knew from church came to the house to see how he was doing. I served coffee and when it was clear they were settling in for the afternoon, I used the opportunity to go for a run. When I returned they were still in the kitchen, deep in conversation, and didn't notice I'd let myself in. My father was out of the room.

"Well, it's about time she moved back to Sydney," I overheard. "She should have done that when her mother was first diagnosed. All this token flying back and forth from Brisbane. Poor man. Whatever she does now will be too little, too late."

I tiptoed back out the front door. Now was definitely a good time to cry.

Mess

*The person who moves mountains begins by
carrying away small stones.*
Chinese proverb

Our ritual conversation each morning of the first week after my mother's funeral went like this:

"When are you going home to Brisbane?" Dad would ask.

"I'm not."

"What about your work?"

"I've resigned."

"Oh." And then a short pause. "When a life starts and ends badly, what happens in between fades into insignificance. I was born without love and now I'm to die without love."

"That isn't being fair to yourself or to Mum," I'd protest. "Life isn't about discrete points and destinations. That would be like saying the only thing that matters in a day is sunrise and sunset. Are you telling me that what we do all day long doesn't count?"

"It doesn't count anymore." He'd retreat back into his Sudoku. Then without looking up he'd ask, "How many Valium tablets would a person need to take if he never wanted to wake up again?"

Without pausing from clearing the table, I would answer, "Regardless of how many tablets he took, he'd wake up in hospital, either having had his stomach pumped or attached to a dialysis machine."

I took to administering my father's medications. It was obvious from his pill boxes that his own dosing was a mess. Actually, *everything* was a mess. My unit in Brisbane had been hastily abandoned in response to a phone call informing me that my mother was drowning in her own fluid. The mail was spilling out of my letterbox because I hadn't had time to get it redirected to Sydney. My speaking engagements had all been postponed indefinitely. My father was in an abyss and I was struggling to stop him from falling ever deeper. My mother's overdue bills, medical reports, X-rays and magazine subscriptions obscured all trace of the coffee table in the lounge room. My inbox held 1703 unread emails. The bedroom I'd reclaimed in my father's home was steeped in dust and carpeted with papers, boxes and amorphous objects. Forgotten food had given rise to new species of emerald and indigo-tinted micro-organisms. A deadly avalanche of expletives swamped unsuspecting telemarketers. Supportive but sadly unacknowledged text messages from friends punctuated the obfuscation like pinholes of light. The anarchy of my surroundings began to infiltrate my mind.

It was time to clean up the mess.

Part II
The Search Begins

I think that only daring speculation can lead us further and not accumulation of facts.

Albert Einstein

Labels

To try where there is little hope is to risk failure.
Not to try at all is to guarantee it.
Unknown

Three years before my mother's death, Dad had been diagnosed with dementia. Although everyone has a vague sense of what dementia is, even the medical community is imprecise and inconsistent in how they define it.

Essentially, dementia is a label indicating progressive loss of mental function affecting at least two areas of cognition, such as memory, concentration, attention, language, problem-solving and social aptitude. The extent of the deficits needs to be such that they interfere with daily life. This makes the term extremely broad. What constitutes interference with daily life? How severe does the interference need to be? Is forgetting the date bad enough? What about losing your keys several times a day? A test called Addenbrooke's Cognitive Examination is a good first step in gauging whether someone needs to be assessed for dementia.

More than 100 types of dementia have been described in the medical literature, each with its own pattern of mental decline. The most common type of dementia in Australia and other developed countries is Alzheimer's Disease (AD), comprising 60 per cent of cases of dementia in older people. Vascular Dementia (VaD) accounts for 15 per cent of cases, and Dementia with Lewy Bodies and Frontotemporal Dementia represent about 5 per cent each. The vast majority of dementias are not hereditary.

Dementia is uncommon in people younger than 60 and is usually the result of alcohol abuse, trauma, Huntington's Disease (an inherited, progressive degenerative disorder that affects muscle coordination) or cerebral infections. An early-onset version of AD can develop before age 50, but it accounts for less than 5 per cent of cases of AD.

In developing countries, AD is less common than VaD. As the name suggests, Vascular Dementia results from blockages in small blood vessels throughout the brain and occurs in up to a third of people in the first year after a stroke. The same things that put people at risk of heart disease also predispose to VaD.

But here's where things get murky. A major risk factor for AD is *also* vascular disease, and some researchers suggest that AD may be a subset of VaD. Dr Alois Alzheimer, who first described AD in 1906, found plaques (collections of a protein called ß-amyloid) scattered throughout the brains of deceased patients with AD. However, when AD develops before age 50, the brain is full of neurofibrillary tangles, rather than plaques. And just to confound the issue further, 30 per cent of people with plaques or tangles in their brains do *not* have dementia! So the role of plaques and tangles in AD is yet to be determined, and we don't know the pathology or cause of Alzheimer's Disease, nor why it is less common in the developing world than in the West.

What we do know is that there are several things we can do to substantially reduce our risk of developing both AD and VaD. What *I* wanted to know was whether such actions could also improve the functioning of people already diagnosed with dementia. Conventional medical doctrine claims that dementia is irreversible and will inevitably worsen with time; I was open to the possibility of conventional medical doctrine being wrong. It wouldn't be the first time this had happened.

Wedding

From the brain, and from the brain only, arise our pleasures, our joys, laughter and jests, as well as our sorrows, pains, griefs and tears.
Hippocrates

My father and I were going to a wedding. Marina, one of my closest friends, had recently become a celebrant. This was her inaugural assignment—her younger brother's wedding. Marina's family were also from the former Yugoslavia (albeit a different "brand" to my family), and her parents were friends of my parents, so I assumed it would be a safe and uplifting experience for my father. He looked very handsome in his best suit, crisp, white cotton shirt, elegant turquoise tie and silver Egyptian cufflinks. But he was taking an inordinately long time in the bathroom, so I knocked on the door.

"Are you OK in there?"

"Yes, all good. I'll be out in a minute."

I waited five minutes. "We have to leave and I still need to blow-dry my hair."

"I'm just dealing with the ant attack on my toothbrush."

"What are you talking about?"

I opened the door and immediately gasped for air. The bathroom was filled with clouds of fly spray, assaulting my nostrils and lungs.

"Get out of here!" I shrieked. "Your clothes will reek of that stuff, if they don't already!"

"I think that's the last of them," he said, taking a final look around.

"Get out! Was it really necessary to do this now?"

"You're always telling me to do things as they come up," he retorted, "to stop putting things off, to avoid having things hang over me. I'm doing exactly what you keep telling me to do and you're *still* whining."

I took a deep breath (outside the bathroom). "Yes, OK, you're right. It's great that you've dealt with the ant attack." I dried my hair in the kitchen.

On the road, we chatted agreeably as I drove.

"What's Marina's brother's name?" asked my father.

"Brian."

"How many guests will be there?"

"I don't know."

"Where's the reception?"

"A function centre in Pyrmont."

"Pyrmont has changed such a lot in the last decade."

"Yes, it has."

"What's Marina's brother's name?"

"Brian."

"How many guests will be there?"

"I don't know."

"Where's the reception?"

"A function centre in Pyrmont."

"Pyrmont has changed such a lot in the last decade."

"Yes, it has."

"What's Marina's brother's name?"

"Brian."

"How many guests will be there?"

"I don't know."

"Where's the reception?"

"A function centre in Pyrmont."

"Pyrmont has changed such a lot in the last decade."

"Yes, it has."

Fortunately, this conversation roundabout ended, as we had a quick run to Pyrmont. On the trip home, my father was more subdued.

"Are you feeling tired?" I ventured.

"Not particularly."

"How did you find it all?"

"OK."

"What's wrong?"

"Marina's parents will never feel alone. They'll always have fulfilment in their lives. They already have three beautiful grandchildren, and no doubt the newlyweds will provide more. I have no-one."

This was becoming a recurring theme between us. We drove home in silence.

Perplexity

We learn more by looking for the answer to a question and not finding it than we do from learning the answer itself.
Lloyd Alexander

Two big questions challenged me: When might dementia not be dementia? And how often do we mistake other conditions for dementia?

A common diagnostic dilemma in geriatric medicine is differentiating dementia from depression. Depression in an older person can manifest as confusion, disorientation, mental dullness and cognitive dysfunction, rather than overt sadness. When depression masquerades as dementia it is given the term "pseudodementia". Could Dad be suffering from that?

Seven years before my mother died, my 87 year-old maternal grandmother became too frail to live alone and moved in with my parents. My mother was working and my father was retired, so for the next four years he became her full-time carer. They were a perfect match. My grandmother was shrewd, observant and diabolically tenacious; my father was phlegmatic, conciliatory and ceaselessly compromising. She gave the orders and he carried them out. She was too unstable on her feet without a walking stick, yet she was able to spring from her chair and stamp her foot whenever anyone contradicted her. My father played along with the game. My grandmother was a chatterbox; my father preferred books to conversation. He became very proficient at disregarding all extraneous noise—particularly human voices— whenever he held a book.

I don't know when Dad first showed signs of patchy, short-term memory loss. Although memory problems are the most common early symptom of dementia, they do not necessarily mean a person has or will progress to dementia. The significance of the memory loss depends on which component of memory is affected: working memory, episodic memory or semantic memory.

Working memory lapses are when we forget people's names or walk into a room and don't remember why we're there. These are more likely to be related to fatigue, anxiety, stress or depression than to dementia. Episodic memory loss is when we repeat ourselves in conversation, not remember what we ate for breakfast, and can't recall recently experienced events. It is more likely to signify early dementia. Semantic memory loss is common in the later stages of dementia, characterised by failing to recall faces, places, words and objects.

It was my father's episodic memory that was most profoundly affected, but my grandmother made it her business to notice and remember everything, so she compensated for his lapses. Dad good-naturedly complained about my grandmother commandeering his life, but my mother and I keenly agreed that it was giving him an enormous sense of worth and purpose. He was very aware of kinship and filial duty and told me that his mother-in-law appreciated him more than his wife.

When my grandmother died at the age of 91, my father must have felt an enormous loss. I say "must have" because no-one spoke about what losing her meant to us. It's highly conceivable Dad became depressed after she passed away. After Granny died, he spent most of his days at home alone, apart from running errands for my mother. He derived his sense of purpose from being there for my mother to debrief. He also went to church on Sundays to pray for us, which was one of the chores my mother assigned to him. He was my mother's buttress. It was during this time that his ability to focus and his capacity to overcome challenges plummeted. He became highly distractible and easily disoriented. He couldn't remember what groceries he was meant to buy. He began taking medication to slow the progression of Alzheimer's Disease.

Watching my father, I wondered whether in some cases dementia might not be a way of protecting ourselves from emotional overload or unbearable mental anguish. Was dementia a way of shielding ourselves from crushing grief, intolerable loneliness, paralysing fear or intractable anxiety? Maybe dementia was the final common pathway for a pain we couldn't face? Dad even spoke about wishing he'd *get* dementia so he could forget his pain—pain that stretched way beyond the loss of his wife and mother-in-law, pain that was anchored in early childhood.

From out of his dementia, I was unable to disentangle his pain, grief, loneliness, fear, confusion, anxiety, apathy, disappointment, shock, inertia, bad habits, stress, poor sleeping, lack of motivation, lack of purpose, loss of hope, loss of confidence, weariness and absence of will to live.

In addition, how much of the principle of "use it or lose it" was at play? When we don't practise something, we don't just forget the skill; the region of the brain responsible for that skill is turned over to doing something else. What that something else is depends on what we do most of the time. It might be a useful function or a bad habit. The principle of use it or lose it governs how the brain develops throughout life. If we start learning a new language, we increase the size of the area of the brain responsible for processing language. If we learn the violin, we activate and enlarge all the areas of the brain related to fine finger movements and appreciation of sound and melody. The reason we don't run out of brain cells for doing new things is that the more proficient we become at something, the more efficiently we use the cells responsible for that function or skill. We end up needing fewer cells to do the job than when we first started, thus freeing up cells to move onto the next new skill. And the more we learn, the better we become at learning.

Conversely, if we don't exercise a particular brain function, the area of the brain associated with that function is allocated to another function.

My father had never been interested in the mundane aspects of life; in this regard, I suspect he was no different to most men of his generation. Cooking, cleaning, tidying, doing the laundry and ironing were of no concern to him, and it was in such activities that he experienced the most visible cognitive loss. He had also learnt to tune out, to switch off from what was going on around him, as a buffer against incessant nagging. Had this contributed to his present difficulty in paying attention when required? What role did his chaotic, cluttered and claustrophobic home environment play? The mess in the house was certainly scrambling *my* brain.

Even severe dehydration can cause mental confusion that resembles dementia. The difference is that mental function reverts to normal when the dehydration is treated. But what if someone had been mildly dehydrated all their life? I had never seen Dad drink water. *Never.* He drank coffee, black tea and soft drinks. And his diet lacked food with a high water content. Could his poor hydration have contributed to his dementia? If that were the case, and if the dehydration was slowly addressed, could his cognitive functioning improve?

Where to begin?

Ironing

*I am not discouraged because every wrong attempt discarded is
another step forward.*
Thomas Edison

Having just completed two huge loads of washing, I was faced
with a large pile of ironing—mostly my father's clothes because
I generally don't buy something if it needs ironing. In particular,
I had to iron the shirt Dad would wear to the opera on Saturday.

For years my mother had subscribed to the opera with a woman
I'd never met. When my mother died, I phoned my mother's
friend and asked if she'd consider going with my father instead.
She agreed on the proviso that, due to her age, we would pick
her up and bring her back home after the performance. I agreed
and found her to be a delightful woman, so I didn't mind playing
chauffeur.

As soon as I pulled out the iron, my father asked what I was
doing.

"The shirt you plan to wear to the opera needs ironing, and your
other clothes from the wash could do with it too."

"You don't need to do the ironing," he informed me. "Your
mother never did the ironing. I take it to a woman who lives a
few blocks away and we pay her to do it."

"Fine with me. But will she get it done by Saturday?"

"Yes, she does it straight away and I sit and chat while she works.
She's by herself most of the time and appreciates the company.
It's a win-win situation."

"You stay there the *whole* time while she does the ironing?" I tried to suppress the glint in my eye. "Even if it's a few *hours'* worth?"

"Well, it's never been a few hours' worth of ironing, but yes, I feel I'm doing my bit of social service if I stay and talk to her."

"How lovely of you—I think that's admirable. Do you want to give her a ring?"

"No, I'll just take it straight there. She's always home."

Wow! A few hours to myself! It was a luxury I hadn't enjoyed in a long time. The list of things I could accomplish flashed before my eyes, and before I knew it I was pulling out as many shirts and shorts of my own that I could crumple up and add to the pile. I managed to fill an entire suitcase.

"There you go," I said, presenting the load to my father. "I'll wheel it to the car for you. And here, take her a box of biscuits. See you later." The door clicked shut and I was on my own. I felt like a kid in a lolly shop.

My bliss was soon shattered. Dad returned within 15 minutes, suitcase in tow.

"Isn't she home?" I asked.

"No. She's in hospital having surgery on her leg. I happened to bump into her daughter, who had arrived to collect the mail, so you'll have to do the ironing after all."

I felt ill. Not only because I'd lost the gift of a few precious hours of solitude, but because I'd wickedly crumpled up my own clothes to add to the workload. Two and a half hours later, I was ready to hurl the iron over the back fence.

Neuroplasticity

How wonderful it is that nobody need wait a single moment
before starting to improve the world.
Anne Frank

For the last decade I've been collating research and speaking about how to keep our brains in peak condition throughout life. During this time, neuroscientists uncovered more about how the brain works than in the centuries of brain research before this. Our knowledge of the brain has exploded and the information is life-changing.

The pivotal discovery was that of neuroplasticity—the ability of the brain to change its anatomical structure, to grow new cells, to make new connections between existing cells, and to re-assign areas of the brain to different functions. The term comes from two words: neuron, or nerve cell, and plastic, meaning malleable or able to be moulded.

The beauty of neuroplasticity is that such changes are not random but are a direct result of each activity the brain performs. Changes in the brain occur in response to what we do, how we behave and even what we think. The implications of this are enormous. It means we can influence how our own brains operate and develop throughout our entire lives. We are *not* destined for inevitable cognitive decline as we age. Instead, we can keep our brains sharp, effective and capable of learning new skills well into our 90s, if we protect our brains from damaging habits and give them ongoing stimulation and appropriate fuel.

The three key elements for a healthy, peak-performing brain are social interaction, physical exercise and mental stimulation. Each of these on its own is highly beneficial, but if we engage in all three for the duration of our lives, the results are extraordinary: a bigger brain, more connections between brain cells, preservation of memory and protection against Alzheimer's Disease. This potential was in direct contrast to what I'd learnt in medical school 20 years ago: that the brain we're born with we're stuck with, and when a part of the brain is damaged or ceases to function, there's little we can do about it. This doctrine was clearly untrue.

We are not passive victims of our genes. Our genes are influenced by our environment and actions. They respond to our attitudes, behaviours, choices, lifestyles and stress levels. Even our thoughts play a role in which genes are expressed and which remain dormant. Our thoughts and beliefs are integral in wiring our brains for optimal health and performance.

There is no quick fix for anything in life, despite what advertising promises. People who are highly educated, intelligent and creative may still end up with dementia. While mentally active people develop dementia at half the rate of people who don't stretch their minds, there are many other factors at play. For the brain to operate at its best and to stay healthy, we need the right nutrition, mental challenges, rest, reward and reinforcement. We also need to take charge of our thinking.

The real-world consequences of neuroplasticity are that no matter how old or young we are, we can:

- Sharpen our thinking
- Improve our concentration and memory
- Increase our capacity for learning and problem-solving
- Expand our creativity
- Tap into brain potential we never knew we had
- Reduce our risk of developing depression, anxiety disorders and dementia
- Perform at our peak on a daily basis
- Achieve far more than we ever thought possible.

Neuroplasticity was my dream come true for my father. I was excited there were so many practical things I could immediately do to improve his mental functioning. Not only that, everything that boosts the brain inevitably also boosts the body. Life was giving me the opportunity to put into intimate practice the very subject I'd been exploring for ten years.

Inspiration

*The secret of success is to start from scratch and
to keep on scratching.*
Dennis Green

I've been inspired by successes with the rehabilitation of stroke patients. For years the medical fraternity believed that a stroke meant lifelong disability. Traditionally, stroke patients were given exercises for four to six weeks. After this time, any improvement plateaued and the patient was essentially told, "That's as good as things will ever get." Most people were left with permanent paralysis of a limb or body part.

In his groundbreaking book, *The Brain that Changes Itself*, Norman Doidge relates the story of a widower named Pedro, who at age 65 had a massive stroke. As a result, Pedro couldn't speak and his face and half his body were paralysed. After the standard four weeks of rehabilitation, Pedro was sent home and his son, George, began a progressive, dedicated effort to retrain his father to walk and talk. Little by little, every day, George encouraged Pedro to use his paralysed limbs. At first Pedro had no strength and could manage only very minimal movement. But with enormous persistence and tenacity, Pedro increased the range and finesse of his movements and his speech, so that by the age of 68 he was able to go back to full-time work. When Pedro died following a heart attack seven years later, his brain was examined at autopsy. It was found to be massively damaged, but the parts that had remained intact after the stroke had re-organised themselves to take over from the parts destroyed by the stroke.

The key to Pedro's remarkable recovery and brain reorganisation was his high motivation and his exposure to incremental exercises that approximated real-life activities. Since then, a treatment program named Constraint-Induced Therapy (CIT) has been developed in the United States to rewire the brains of stroke patients and restore the use of their paralysed limbs. CIT is based on the practice of constraining the good limb and forcing the patient to use the stroke-affected limb, one tiny step at a time. The therapy is very intense, involving constant repetition of drills six hours a day for several weeks, but the results are astounding: 80 per cent of stroke patients substantially improve, even if it's been *decades* since their stroke.

The message is that if there's a demand for something, the brain will find a way to achieve it. Given the appropriate stimulation and training, the brain can restructure itself and find new ways to perform lost functions. **Use it or lose it; train it and regain it.**

Why couldn't the same principle be applied to memory impairment and cognitive deficits? As long as Dad was able to comprehend what I asked him to do, I could give him graded exercises to rebuild his mental functioning. At the same time, I would give him the best environment and lifestyle to boost his overall brain performance.

The literature on brain retraining indicates that the best results are achieved when the training is:

- Related to activities of daily life—I would have to give my father chores and drills around the house that had a practical purpose and didn't just appear to be random exercises.
- Done in increments—each small, successive achievement needed to be acknowledged and rewarded.
- Concentrated and continued from one day to the next.

It was time for some tough love.

Threshold

Brain cells create ideas. Stress kills brain cells.
Stress is not a good idea.
Frederick Saunders

Much as I needed to make sure my father persisted with his training from one day to the next, it was equally important that he didn't find the exercises stressful. I felt he needed to be stretched just enough to jolt him out of his apathy, but not to the point of anxiety. **Fun, not force**, was the goal.

A bit of stress is not necessarily a bad thing because it can actually fire us up. This is known as eustress. But once our stress levels exceed a certain threshold, technically referred to as our allostatic load, our performance and ability to learn start to plummet. One reason for this is that acute stress diverts blood from the frontal lobe higher centres of intelligence to the primitive reflex parts of the brain in preparation for a fight or flight, whether or not we end up in a fight or flight. That was why I couldn't remember an answer while sitting in an exam room, but it came to me as soon as I walked out the door and the stress dissipated.

Worse still are the effects of chronic stress because they switch off the production of new brain cells and can even kill neurons in the hippocampus, which is the brain's memory and learning warehouse. "Hippocampus" comes from the Latin for seahorse because the structure resembles a seahorse in size and shape. It is in the middle region of the brain, with a mirror image of itself in the right and left hemispheres. The hippocampus plays a vital role in converting short-term into long-term memories and in orienting us in time and place. It is particularly sensitive to the stress hormone cortisol because it's generously endowed with cortisol receptors. Prolonged stress can also drag us into depression. Given that stress profoundly affects mood regulation and immediate and long-term brain function, it was definitely to be avoided by my father.

Boat

*A lot of people ask me if I were shipwrecked, and could only
have one book, what would it be? I always say,*
How to Build a Boat.
Stephen Wright

The brain and mind can be thought of as a large boat, complete with captain and crew, sailing the ocean blue.

The captain makes the decisions and gives the orders, which the loyal crew follow. Without a captain, the boat would be directionless. Without a crew, the day-to-day running of the boat would be impossible. The crew know their role and don't need the captain to tell them how to do their job or to remind them of their job on a daily basis. They're very well trained. The captain only notifies the crew if he or she wants something to change and takes charge whenever leadership is required. As for the boat, it needs to be kept in good nick and fuelled on a regular basis.

The captain, the crew and the boat form a single, interdependent unit, each party influencing the other two. If the captain and crew don't do their job properly, the boat can get damaged and end up in disrepair. If the boat is damaged, the journey is more arduous; in particular, rough seas are more difficult to handle. If the captain is apathetic, incompetent or drunk, there is an absence of leadership. And if the captain and crew are in constant disagreement, they won't get very far.

How does this relate to the brain and mind? The captain represents the conscious mind; the crew represent the subconscious mind; the boat is the brain; and the ocean is life.

The conscious mind is the thinking part of ourselves. It sets goals, makes decisions and interprets experiences. The subconscious mind is the part of ourselves beneath our conscious awareness that keeps us alive and running. It's what keeps our hearts pumping, our lungs expanding and our hair growing. We don't consciously say to ourselves, "Pump, breathe, grow!"—these things are handled subconsciously, through the autonomic nervous system. The number one priority of the subconscious mind is our survival: physical, emotional and psychological. This is why our subconscious plays a powerful role in dictating behaviour. It prioritises our emotional wellbeing over our conscious wants. It's why sometimes we consciously think we want one thing, but still end up doing another. One reason that diets don't work is they don't address subconscious issues that may be at play. We always sabotage our efforts if the subconscious pay-offs for not changing override the conscious desire to lose weight. Finally, the brain is the vessel through which our conscious and subconscious minds operate.

Based on the analogy of boat, captain and crew, I drew up the following plan for boosting Dad's brain.

1.   Don't damage the boat.

On day one in medical school, I was taught *Primum non nocere*—"First do no harm". No boat owner would knowingly damage his boat, so it follows that no human would knowingly damage his brain. Apart from the obvious injury caused by falling off ladders and falling into illegal drugs, things that harm the brain and reduce our cognitive abilities include smoking, stress, sleep deprivation, soft drinks, sedentary lifestyles, excessive alcohol, junk food, high blood pressure, obesity, loneliness, pessimism and negative self-talk. Goal number one is to avoid these damaging entities.

2.   Dock the boat in stimulating surroundings.

Our brain function improves in every measurable way when we find ourselves in environments that are mentally, physically and socially stimulating. **Adventure prevents dementia!**

3. Fuel it the finest.

Our dietary choices affect not only the health of our bodies but also the health of our brains. In fact our brains consume *one fifth* of all the nutrients and kilojoules we ingest. What we eat has a significant impact on our neurotransmitters (chemicals that carry messages between neurons across synapses), energy levels, alertness, mood and cognitive functioning.

4. Keep the cargo light.

Excess visceral (abdominal) fat is a major risk factor for dementia. As a rough guide, a healthy waist circumference for a man is under 94 cm and for a woman is under 80 cm.

5. Run the motor.

Without physical exercise our brains waste away as much as our muscles waste away. Exercise actually induces the growth of new brain cells.

6. Learn the ropes and keep on learning.

Having a good education and engaging in lifelong, active learning help to protect us from dementia and contribute to our developing "cognitive reserve". This reserve acts as a buffer against mental decline as we age.

7. Sail to new shores.

Boredom and monotony are poisonous to our brains. We need to get out there, get exploring and get out of our comfort zones. We need to sail to new shores to find riches outside our usual boundaries. We need to change our routines, do things differently and give ourselves ongoing challenges.

8. Use it or lose it.

This applies to every function of the brain and body, from studying to socialising to sex. In order to maintain our capacity for learning new skills, we need to *engage* in learning new skills on a regular basis. In order to become creative, inventive and resourceful, we need to give ourselves tasks that require creativity, inventiveness and resourcefulness. In order to have a good memory, we need to make a conscious effort to pay attention. In order to remain socially adept, we need to remain socially active.

9. Train it and regain it.

If we lose a specific brain function, all is not lost. Progressive, persistent, goal-focused practice can help us regain the lost function.

10. Charge the battery.

Stilling the mind is as important as stimulating the mind. Getting adequate sleep and pressing the pause button on our mind chatter are essential for peak performance on a day-to-day basis, as well as preservation of brain function as we age.

11. Connect with fellow travellers.

Lifelong social interaction and meaningful connection with others is vital for a healthy brain.

12. Choose the destination.

The brain is a teleological device—it is fed by having goals to strive for and aspirations to work towards. The clearer we are about where we want to go and what we want to achieve, the more effective the brain is in accomplishing the required tasks. This is analogous to the captain giving the crew clear instructions about where they're going and what is expected of them.

13. Command the crew.

Having decided on what we want, we need to direct our self-talk to support our goals. Our internal dialogue is a constant stream of instructions to the subconscious mind. Uplifting, solution-focused self-talk switches on brain cell activity; negative, discouraging self-talk dampens it.

14. Communicate gratitude.

When we think about what we're thankful for, we wire our brains to *continue finding* things to be thankful for. Our brains are designed so that we see whatever we're looking for. We are never objective, even when we make a concerted effort to be so.

Subjectivity always enters our perceptions. We don't see things as *they* are; we see things as *we* are. Therefore, by regularly reflecting on things that we're grateful for, we construct a filter through which we see the world and we create more experiences for which to feel grateful.

15. Practise perfectly.

When we practise a skill in our imaginations, the same neurons are firing *as if we were performing the skill in real life*! If we see ourselves executing a task perfectly in the mind's eye, we become better at it in the real world because every mental rehearsal increases the efficiency of electrical transmissions between the involved nerve cells. Mental practice turbocharges our progress.

16. Bon voyage!

Enjoy the journey! Get excited about where you're going. Passion, enthusiasm and excitement are the most powerful brain fuels of all. The word enthusiasm comes from the Greek *entheos,* meaning "to be divinely inspired or possessed by a god". Ralph Waldo Emerson observed, "Nothing great has ever been achieved without enthusiasm."

To my plan, I added four mantras to preserve my own sanity:

1. **Fun not force**

2. **Feedback not failure**

3. **Curious not critical**

4. **Direction not perfection**

Nature

Whoever loves and understands a garden will find
contentment within.
Chinese proverb

Our physical environment influences the structure and function of our brains. We need to **dock the boat in stimulating surroundings**.

Spending as little as five minutes a day in nature, in a park or garden, measurably improves mood and self-esteem, particularly in the young and those suffering from a mental illness. Adding a view of water and some physical exercise confers even greater benefit.

Nature also helps us concentrate. People who live surrounded by trees perform better in attention tests than people whose homes are surrounded by concrete. A possible reason is that natural surroundings tend to capture our attention and give us a rest from deliberately focusing on specific tasks.

One of my father's most debilitating symptoms was distractibility and difficulty focusing. It was a major contributing factor to his memory loss; the information reaching his brain was indistinct and contaminated with static, so he couldn't register things. Consequently, he couldn't remember them. Before I could begin specific work on his memory, Dad's brain needed to relearn how to focus, so every afternoon for half an hour my father and I wandered around our leafy garden or went to a nearby park.

The other major benefit of this was exposure to sunshine, our best source of vitamin D. In a six-year study of 858 adults aged 65 years and older, those with the lowest blood levels of vitamin D were 60 per cent more likely than those with normal vitamin D levels to show signs of general cognitive decline. They were also 31 per cent more likely to have difficulty with planning, organising and prioritising. This study was confirmed by data from more than 3000 elderly Americans that showed a dose-dependent relationship between vitamin D deficiency and symptoms of Alzheimer's Disease: the greater the vitamin D deficiency, the greater the decline in cognitive function. As little as 10 minutes of sunshine a day or a total of one hour per week (without sunscreen) gives most people adequate levels of vitamin D. This is particularly important during winter.

The light available in the home and workplace also has an impact on the brain. Bright lights increase both alertness and ability to pay attention. A US study of elderly people in residential care found that in homes with bright lighting, residents had better cognition, mood and sleeping habits compared with those where the lighting was dim.

My parents' home was dark and overwhelmingly cluttered. My father's new, first chore for the day was to pull up the blinds, draw aside the tan curtains and open the russet, wooden back door. Then we would sit down to breakfast.

Train Window

Ageing seems to be the only available way to live a long life.
Daniel François Esprit Auber

For as long as I could remember, Dad's morning staple consisted of Scotch Finger biscuits dipped in instant coffee. I'd been campaigning against this for 20 years—it was finally time to rectify the situation.

"I can't find my breakfast," my father said. "Do you know where all the biscuits have gone?"

"Your breakfast is right here," I smiled, handing him a bowl of fresh berries with natural yoghurt. "I've also boiled some eggs for you. What would you prefer?" **Fuel it the finest.**

"No thanks, I prefer the usual."

"This is so much better for you. You'll think more sharply, feel more energetic, succumb to fewer infections and function better all round."

"No thanks."

"Research has found that eating berries or eggs for breakfast is associated with better mental functioning than eating something sugary like biscuits."

"I've managed to survive 78 years without berries or eggs for breakfast. Changing what I eat at this stage of life isn't going to make one iota of difference."

"Yes, it absolutely *will* make a difference!" I insisted. "It's *never* too late to experience improvement in your health and well-being, particularly when it comes to your brain. That

1.4 kilogram wrinkled lump of grey matter constitutes less than 2 per cent of your body weight but it uses 20 per cent of your blood supply and 20 per cent of your energy, and it generates 20 per cent of your heat. It consumes a disproportionate amount of your resources. Older rats fed blueberries, strawberries and spinach leaves learn new tasks much quicker than rats fed the usual rat diet."

"Now you're calling me a rat?"

"Beagle dogs fed fruit and vegetables," I continued, "learn new tricks faster than dogs with poor dietary habits, even in old age. So you *can* teach an old dog new tricks."

"I'm not a circus animal and I don't want to learn new tricks."

"Stop being so obstinate. Rat, dog or human, what you eat affects your memory, your mood, your concentration, your ability to learn and your decision-making skills."

Dad was now opening the kitchen cupboards. "What are you doing?" I asked.

"I'm looking for my biscuits."

"You're not listening to me."

"No, *you're* not listening to *me*! I *don't care* about better mental functioning. What's the point?"

"I'm sick of hearing you say 'what's the point?' There's no point to anything if we don't want there to be. There's no point to life except to live. So while you're alive, get on with the business of living in the best possible state you can!"

I was losing patience. My fear of losing Dad soon after losing Mum rendered me incapable of empathising with him. Fear is a blinding force; as is grief. My father looked at me as though I were from another planet.

"In the best possible state? I am in *no* state for anything. What's happened to your philosophy of 'live and let live'? That's what you used to say to your mother whenever she tried to impose her will on *you*. Now you're trying to impose *your* will on *me*. You're being hypocritical."

"This is different," I countered. "If I were to live and let you live the way you wanted, you'd soon be dead."

"Maybe that's what I want."

"I can't let that happen."

"What's the point of sustaining a life that's devoid of any meaning, purpose, love, joy? Everything that makes life worth living has been taken away from me."

"I'm still here."

He raised his eyebrows at me mistrustfully.

"Then why don't you make yourself useful and prescribe me enough Valium, so I never wake up again?"

"It's not your time to go."

"It wasn't your mother's time to go and she's gone."

We sat in silence staring at the fruit salad. It had become a symbol of life's cruelty, of upheaval, of unwanted reform, of uncertainty.

I tried not to sound robotic. "Life is never going to feel worse than it feels right now. It's called grief." He continued to stare in silence. I pressed on. "The fact that you're alive means there's something left for you to do in this world."

"Your mother still had so much left to do. Nothing makes sense. I'm the man; I should have died first. And if gender wasn't enough of a warranty, I'm nine years older than your mother. That should have been sufficient margin for error. I was never supposed to bury my wife."

"Life doesn't always make sense," I lamely responded.

He disregarded my interruption. "I can't understand why she was taken away from me. What did I do to deserve such enormous punishment?"

"I don't believe suffering is dished out as punishment; it is never 'deserved'. Suffering looks to me like an interplay of events and reactions that we're not always able to comprehend. Whenever I can't fathom something, I imagine life being like a train ride. I'm sitting in my carriage looking out the window. I can see only as far as the window frame allows. I got on the train at a certain point on its route, and at some other point I'll get off. Sometimes what I see outside the window is beautiful and I feel happy. Sometimes what I see shocks and saddens me. Sometimes I understand how what I'm looking at has come about because of what I've seen on my journey so far. Sometimes I'm totally baffled. Sometimes I think that what I'm looking at is ugly, but I find as the journey continues, the ugliness transforms into something unexpectedly grand. But at the time, because of that window frame, I couldn't know what was ahead. It doesn't mean the ugliness never happened or wasn't painful, but had it not been for the pain, I'd have missed out on an experience that deepened my appreciation of life in ways I never imagined possible.

"That train ride is life. When I step onto the train I am born. The window allows me to see only the present moment. I'm able to remember what I see along the way but can never be sure what's ahead. I'll never see the entire picture. I'll never be able to stand on the roof of the train and get a 360 degree view, so my judgements will always be based on a limited perspective."

I looked at my grieving father. "I'm not trying to negate how you're feeling, only to say that things change with time and neither you nor I have any idea what lies in store for us."

Witness

Age wrinkles the body. Quitting wrinkles the soul.
General Douglas MacArthur

"You don't need me. You haven't needed a father in a long time."

"But I *want* a father."

"Why would you want the decrepit remains of a man like me?"

"Do you remember how I spent a year in Japan as a Rotary Exchange student when I was 18 years old?"

"Of course I do."

"I don't know if things have changed since I was there, but a younger person encountering an older person always had to bow lower and longer."

"What does this have to do with needing me?"

"Just hear me out. Within the home, the oldest member of the family, usually a grandfather, got the first dip in the hot bath every night. Even as an esteemed foreign guest, I had to wait my turn, based on my age. There was a pervading air of 'this older person is important', even if it was 'only' as an observer of the life around them. And I remember thinking back then, 'It's really comforting to have a witness in life, especially someone you care about and want to make proud.' My experience in Japan was all the more meaningful because I was sharing it with you through letters and phone calls. Because I'd be able to show you the photos when I came home. Because I'd give you the experience of a tea ceremony on my return. My life has changed and I no longer need to show you what I did at school, but we're never too old to have our lives deepened by the presence of a witness. There is value in you *being* here. I want you here. Got that?"

I left the room before he could reply.

Expectations

Argue for your limitations, and sure enough, they are yours.
Richard Bach

Dad did not fit the stereotypical picture of dementia, as a doddery old man who wandered about aimlessly, mistaking me for the local pharmacist. However, I couldn't deny that he fulfilled the diagnostic criteria of Alzheimer's Disease: insidious onset of short-term memory impairment, inability to follow through with complex tasks, disorientation with respect to time and place, and difficulty with decision making, planning and organising.

One evening, I left the house and instructed Dad to heat up his dinner in the microwave oven while I was gone. When I returned, everything seemed to be in order. Two days later, I discovered his untouched meal in the microwave. He'd heated it up as instructed, but then forgotten to take it out and eat it. I cried for a long time.

Fortunately, he was unaware of the diagnosis but he was sometimes cognisant of being forgetful. He knew that he frequently misplaced his keys but wasn't aware that he asked me 20 times a day (sometimes more) what day of the week it was.

My father completed his degree in electrical engineering at Belgrade Technical University but had always been fascinated by archaeology, mythology, ancient history and theology. Consequently he was extremely well read. He also appreciated classical literature and at one stage had been fluent in French. His favourite subject was maths and he could spend hour after hour, day after day, solving Sudoku puzzles. He claimed to be an introvert but was a great raconteur. I loved listening to his stories, both as a child and as an adult. He had a playful sense of humour. He loved antiques. He still read the Serbian newspaper every day.

Dad's intelligence and education, coupled with my mother's dominance, extroversion and all-round competence, masked his declining cognitive function. Even *I* forgot about it when we were engaged in a philosophical discussion.

"You can't understand me because you're in the prime of your life," was his favourite opener. "Old age is no fun. Joints creak, eyesight and hearing diminish, teeth fall out and everything I attempt to do is exhausting. I have naught left to contribute and there's absolutely nothing to look forward to. I'm just a waste of resources."

"Then why is medical science continually trying to prolong life?" I quizzed him.

"Because the scientists doing the research are all young and naïve. It sounds great in theory to live a long time, but when you reach old age you realise you've entered a detention centre."

"It doesn't have to be that way," I objected. "Attitudes to ageing are culturally and economically driven. Because we live in a fast-paced, consumer-based society that values productivity and profit above community and connection, old age has lost its status. Yes, ageing is accompanied by physical, hormonal and psychological changes, but these don't render a human being incapable or worthless. It all depends on your values.

"Western culture values financial success. And financial success is largely achieved through selling more things to more people. You can sell more things to young people because they're more vulnerable to messages on billboards. They're still trying to establish their place in the world and still discovering what makes them happy. Their concerns revolve around 'fitting in', creating the 'right' image and visible accomplishment. This makes them a great target for anyone trying to sell anything. Buy this and it'll make you happy. But older people know better. They know the things that make us happy aren't *things*. Also, by the time they reach old age, most of them have everything they need for practical survival—a fridge, furniture, toaster—so they have little reason to spend money, other than on perishables. This makes older people very unattractive to big business."

"I'm equally unattractive to myself," Dad chimed in.

"That's only because we live in a culture that fails to recognise all the things you have to offer. Why is it that we tend to focus on what we lose over time rather than what we gain?"

"I know what you're going to say: that we gain experience, understanding and wisdom." He rolled his eyes. "What use is any of it if there's no goal or purpose to put it towards?"

"You can put your experience, understanding and wisdom towards *finding* a goal or purpose."

"Your mother gave me purpose. Everything else is meaningless."

"Sorry, I don't buy that. It wasn't Mum's job to give you a purpose. That's *your* job."

I knew I was sounding harsh, but the terror of losing him had taken root again and sucked the compassion out of me. Lately I was always operating in matter-of-fact mode, to give the impression of being on top of things. I never allowed Dad to see me upset or grieving, for fear of it dragging him down even further. In hindsight, he, too, just needed me to be "real". How quickly I'd forgotten the lesson I'd learnt by my dying mother's bedside.

"I've retired," Dad said.

"Retirement wasn't created because people above a certain age were incompetent or unable to work," I continued. "Retirement was a response to the Great Depression. Governments wanted to reduce unemployment, so they gave older people an incentive to stop working, in order to open up jobs for people entering the workforce. Unfortunately, the retirement age has created the perception that it's the age of physical and mental decline but this isn't biologically true. In certain rural regions of Japan, as well as in China and Africa, people work for as long as they can, regardless of age. They maintain their sense of value and belonging until the day they die. In Native American cultures, important community decisions were traditionally the domain of a circle of elders whose wisdom was honoured and heeded."

"What galaxy are you from? How can you say that we don't experience physical and mental decline as we age?"

"We experience *change*—not necessarily *decline*. Decline is a value judgement."

"Euphemisms don't change facts."

"Actually, they do. How we label things, the meaning we assign to change, determines how we behave and how we respond to that change. We live into our expectations of life. If we think we aren't capable of something, we don't attempt it or at best we make a half-hearted effort. If I'm doing something I believe I'm able to do and I come up against an obstacle, I view it as an interesting challenge. I usually enjoy it and get a feeling of satisfaction from working through it. But if I don't believe I'm capable of something, an obstacle feels like an insurmountable problem and I moan and groan about it until I convince myself that 'it wasn't meant to be, so I may as well give up'. We don't see things as they really are, but as we expect them to be.

"There's a well known experiment in which school teachers were advised that a group of average to below-average students were actually gifted, high performers. By the end of term, it became a self-fulfilling prophecy. The teachers treated the students as exceptionally talented, seeing any mistakes as learning opportunities and instilling in their students the belief that they were highly competent—and that's exactly what they became. We need to treat ourselves in the same way. **Command the crew.**"

"Nurturing talent isn't the same as defying our biological clock," my father insisted. He was getting frustrated with what he saw as my Pollyanna attitude.

"I'm not trying to defy your biological clock, I'm trying to work *with* it. Fundamentally, we have a use-it-or-lose-it body and brain. Both your muscles and your brain atrophy with disuse. The more actively you engage your brain and the more ways you use your brain, the bigger, more complex and more effective it can become. It's the same as if you go to the gym and pump iron, you'll build bigger and stronger muscles."

He remained unimpressed. "But there will always be a loss of brain cells as we age, regardless of what we do."

"The loss is minimal," I clarified. "With the current techniques for counting and measuring brain cells, we've found that the ageing process is *not* accompanied by the loss of a significant number of brain cells. Our brains do not shrink markedly with age, unless we consistently consume more than 20 grams of alcohol per day—that's two standard drinks, so you have nothing to worry about on that count.

"Declining brain function is due to years of inadequate nutrition, insufficient physical exercise and not enough appropriate stimulation. Also, because we expect things to go downhill as we age, we attempt less, we slow down and we put fewer demands on our brains. This causes areas of the brain that are not being used to begin shutting down, further confirming the belief that we aren't as sharp and quick as we used to be. So we attempt even less, we lose confidence and the result is a self-perpetuating, downward spiral.

"If you forget something at the age of 20, you think nothing of it. You ignore it and move on. If you forget something at the age of 60, you call it a 'senior moment', thereby reinforcing the belief that your memory is declining with age."

Dad shrugged.

"The only reason you find what I say heretical is that our entire culture magnifies the perceived deficits that come with age. The entire race—or Western society at least—needs to change its mindset."

He shrugged again. Was I becoming a nag? I shuddered at the possibility. I hated the thought of lecturing my father, but I didn't know how else to deal with what I perceived to be his defeatism. I tried to lighten the tone.

"People *pay* me to give them this information, and all you can do is shrug! I could be charging you for this."

"I could be charging you for rent."

"I could be charging you for housekeeping!"

"I could be charging you for the hire of my car." He remained exasperatingly composed.

"You don't stand a chance of winning this game," I declared.

"That depends how far back in time you want to play."

I elected not to pursue the issue.

"Besides," he continued, "*you* create work for *me*."

"Excuse me?"

"When you cook, you use a lot more utensils and pots and pans than your mother ever did and you make me do the washing up."

"Speaking of which …"

"Yeah, yeah, I'm onto it."

Research

*If I'd known how old I was going to be, I'd have taken
better care of myself.*
Adolph Zukor

OK, so maybe berries, yoghurt and eggs were a bit ambitious for day one. I decided to try the Gradual Transition Approach (GTA) instead.

"I know you like biscuits for breakfast, so I've bought you some new ones to try."

"What kind of biscuits?" Dad eyed me suspiciously. "Just try them."

"Are they good for dunking into coffee?"

"Um … yes. But why don't you put them into a bowl instead? It's less messy that way."

I placed two Weet-Bix in a bowl. "What about if you have them with milk instead of coffee?"

"No thanks." He poured his coffee over the Weet-Bix.

"OK, whatever you prefer."

I tried to eat my own breakfast as casually as possible. I didn't want to look like a cat eyeing a mouse hole.

"I prefer the old biscuits. These aren't as sweet."

I pounced. "Then why not add a banana? That will give it sweetness."

"Why not just add sugar?"

"A banana will give it a better flavour as well as sweetness. Not to mention providing you with vitamin B6, vitamin C, potassium, fibre and manganese."

"The old biscuits made for a lot less fuss. You like to complicate life, don't you?"

"Not complicate life, *improve* life. Eating bananas can help prevent high blood pressure and protect against hardening of your arteries."

"Does every conversation with you have to sound like a lecture? No wonder you can't hold down a relationship. It's driving me nuts and *I* have the luxury of forgetting half of what you say."

Basics

Failure is success if we learn from it.
Malcolm Forbes

Increasing the fruit and vegetable component of my father's diet proved more challenging than I'd imagined. There is no word for "vegetarian" in the original Serbian language. A corruption of the English word has recently appeared in Serbian to reflect a small number of young converts, but on the whole, vegetables are just garnish to meat. This should have given me a clue to the resistance I might encounter. Not that I was trying to convert my father to vegetarianism. I only wanted to shift the balance from 100 per cent carnivore plus dairy products to 50 per cent herbivore, again using the Gradual Transition Approach (GTA).

Dad loved macaroni cheese, so I made it my first target.

"This is different to the way your mother made it."

"Is it?"

"What are these lumpy, white bits?"

"Cauliflower." I thought by hiding a white vegetable in the macaroni cheese, I might slip it under his radar.

"Cauliflower?"

"Yes, I had some in the fridge so I thought I'd use it up."

"How does cauliflower come to take up residence in our fridge unless you make a deliberate effort to buy it? This was premeditated."

"But do you like it?"

"I'll eat it."

The next time I made macaroni cheese, I added peas and broccoli as well as cauliflower—optimistic, I know.

"What's with the green stuff in the macaroni cheese?"

"You weren't overly keen on the cauliflower, so I thought I'd add some other vegetables to dilute it."

"I don't suppose it crossed your mind to leave the cauliflower out altogether?"

"Do you like it better than with cauliflower alone?"

"I like it better with cheese alone. But I'll eat it."

These were two of my *success* stories. (Thinly sliced brussels sprouts concealed between layers of potato bake was another of my triumphs.) But more often than not, it was a mammoth effort to get him to eat anything, carnivorous or otherwise. Had my father been overweight, his lack of appetite wouldn't have worried me. Excess fat around internal organs (called visceral fat) can double the risk of dementia by age 75. As can type 2 diabetes and high blood pressure in midlife. **Keep the cargo light.**

But Dad was bordering on underweight and he had little enough energy as it was. Most days I'd have to contend with one or all of the following: "I'm not hungry. Why do I have to eat if I'm not hungry? I don't want anything, thanks. Haven't I already eaten today? I have a tummy ache. The effort it takes me to eat probably uses up more calories than I consume." (I could have said the same for the effort it took me to coax him into eating.) "How about you take a break from cooking today? I'm feeling nauseous. You place too much importance on nutrition. Give it a rest."

But his best line was: "I had lunch while you were doing the washing." I knew this to be blatantly untrue. I was aware of exactly what was in the fridge and in all the cupboards, and nothing was ever missing. When I asked him what he'd eaten he could never remember. I didn't know whether he was lying or he actually believed that he'd eaten, as a result of his memories from previous days merging; I came to think it was the latter. Because his brain was not registering hunger, the only explanation he could think of was that he must have eaten already.

Perhaps I'd have an easier time, I thought, if I went back to basics and simply asked him to choose his favourite fruit and vegetable, something he'd enjoy. Whenever I asked him what he wanted to eat, his answer would invariably be, "Nothing." Maybe I needed to narrow it down for him.

"I know you're not big on fruit, but how about eating just one piece of fruit a day? I'll get you any fruit you want. I'll even peel it for you." Dad actively avoided anything that required a shred of effort on his part. "What's something you really like? What's your favourite fruit?"

"Quinces."

I searched his face for a sign that he was joking. "Are you serious?"

"Of course I'm serious."

"But you can't eat quinces raw. Quinces would have to be the only fruit on the planet that have to be cooked to render them edible."

"Yes, my grandmother made the best stewed quinces," he reminisced. "She said they were a symbol of love and fertility, which is why Croats traditionally plant a quince tree when a baby is born. And some Bible scholars suggest that it was a quince, not an apple, that the serpent offered Eve in the Garden of Eden."

"Thanks for the history lesson. How about the recipe?"

"My grandmother started cooking in the morning and they'd be ready by dinner."

"Tell me you're pulling my leg."

The phone rang; it was a medical practice where I occasionally did locum work.

"Are you able to work for us next Wednesday? One of our doctors will be away."

"Only if you can give me a recipe for stewed quinces."

"Stewed quinces?"

"Yes."

"But they take nine hours of slow cooking. Don't you have enough to do without adding basting quinces to your day?"

"I'm trying to get some fibre into my father."

"What about a banana?"

"Just email me the quince recipe."

Peel, core and cut 3 quinces into eighths. Drop into water with juice of half a lemon to stop them discolouring. Place into a deep casserole dish with seeds of one vanilla bean and 6 strips of lemon zest. Sprinkle over one tablespoon of cinnamon and one tablespoon of raw sugar. Cover with lid and put into 180 degree Celsius oven for one hour, then turn down to 80 degrees Celsius for 8 hours. Turn once or twice during that time to keep coated.

I have to admit, they were delicious. And Dad even had a second helping—we were on our way!

Assumptions

It is through science that we prove but
through intuition that we discover.
Jules H. Poincaré

The tyranny of memory loss was that my father felt I kept him in the dark. "You always spring things on me without warning!" was a frequent complaint, even though I always warned him a dozen times.

But memory loss had its upside. Dad and I never ran out of things to talk about because we'd recycle the same conversation several times a week, if not every day. It also meant that in that first, tormented week after my mother died, I was able to negotiate one more day of life for him, every day. He didn't remember that I'd asked him to make me the same promise the previous morning: to give me just one more day of his life. "Wait and see what the view out of the train window is like tomorrow," I'd say. "Then we'll talk again."

My father's capacity for erudite discourse was in stark contrast to his inability to function on a practical level. I searched for tasks he could succeed in, to build up his confidence and sense of self-mastery. It was very much a case of trial and error.

The first time I took on a day's work at the local GP practice, I made sure Dad had everything he needed for the eight hours I'd be away. I'd bought him a brand new Sudoku book; lunch was clearly labelled and placed on the top shelf of the fridge; and I'd composed a short shopping list, to get him out of the house for an hour. His first phone call came only minutes after I'd arrived at work.

"Where did you put my South African ostrich skin belt with the Australian opal buckle?"

"Sorry?"

"Your mother bought if for me and it was always in the brown cupboard in the back room. It's not there now."

"I didn't know you owned an ostrich skin belt with an opal buckle. In fact, I didn't know anyone owned an ostrich skin belt with an opal buckle. Can we continue this conversation when I get home?" The second phone call came less than an hour later.

"Why do you keep taking my clothes from one cupboard and putting them in another? I can't find anything any more because you keep rearranging things. Stop it. It's very frustrating."

I had done no such thing. "OK, I'll stop it."

The third phone call came shortly before lunch. "I'm so sorry, I went shopping but I wasn't able to buy a pineapple. I bought everything else but I was afraid of getting a pineapple in case it was the wrong one."

"How can you buy the *wrong* pineapple?"

"Well, you wrote down that you wanted a ripe one, but I couldn't tell which were ripe and which weren't."

"That's fine, don't worry about it. It wouldn't have mattered if you'd bought an unripe one because it would have ripened in a few days. But next time we go shopping together, I'll show you how to choose a ripe pineapple. Thanks for buying all the other things."

"What time will you be home?"

"Shortly after five o'clock."

Ninety minutes later. "What time will you be home?"

"Shortly after five o'clock."

And then at four o'clock, "Is there any cake in the house?"

"Not unless you baked one."

"A Serbian woman feels naked if she doesn't have cake in the house."

"I'm comfortable with my nudity."

"But what am I to offer a visitor if someone drops by?"

"I'll be home soon, so we'll sort it out then."

"What time is soon?"

"Shortly after five o'clock."

I was relieved to arrive home. "How was your lunch?" I asked.

"It was pretty boring."

"How so? It was last night's leftovers. You said you liked it last night."

"All you left me was broccoli."

"And other vegetables and a piece of meat, each in its own container. All you needed to do was dish them out onto a plate and heat them in the microwave."

"There was only broccoli."

I opened the fridge. The broccoli had been eaten but the meat and other vegetables hadn't been touched. "Why didn't you eat the meat and vegetables?"

"You only labelled the broccoli box. How was I supposed to know you wanted me to eat the meat and other vegetables as well?"

"The three boxes were sitting on top of each other and the label was on the top box, meaning the entire *pile* was your lunch."

"I don't make assumptions. It's the quickest way to get into trouble. You labelled one box of food and I ate one box of food."

This time I was the one who sighed. Dad wasn't playing games with me; he genuinely believed that if I'd intended him to eat what was in all three boxes, I'd have labelled all three boxes. I had no trouble getting him to eat dinner that night—for once he was actually hungry.

Progress

The only way to discover the limits of the possible is to go beyond them into the impossible.
Arthur C. Clarke

With time I developed strategies for reducing the possibility of my father misinterpreting the instructions I left for him when I went out. Usually the easiest thing was to drag my father with me everywhere I had to go, including on dates with Daniel, my unbelievably tolerant boyfriend of 12 months.

Dad, Dan and I dined out together, went to the movies together, saw musicals, dance performances and stage plays together, or spent quiet evenings at home together. Whenever Dan was around, my father was at his brightest, most animated and most wakeful. He always outlasted us. The evening would invariably conclude with Dad cheerfully watching me wave Dan goodbye.

On the rare occasions I left the house without Dad, I placed a note on the kitchen table stating what time I'd be home. I reasoned that this would halve the number of phone calls I received while I was out. Not so. My father would either forget about or lose the note, so I attached a whiteboard to the fridge and trained him to look at it before he reached for the phone. Every piece of food for my father was separately labelled, and I included assembly instructions for every meal or put everything on a plate in the fridge myself. Every light switch and every lamp had a pink Post-it note stuck to it—TURN ME OFF.

The Gradual Transition Approach (GTA) was effective in giving Dad a degree of independence in daily living. One of my proudest days was when he made his own way to Manly to visit his longstanding friend, Marko. We built up to this feat in four stages, over a period of a month, with several practice runs each week.

Stage I: Together we walked from home to the train station (about 20 minutes), bought tickets, caught the train to Circular Quay, went to Wharf 3, took the Manly ferry across Sydney Harbour, and were met by Marko at the bus-stop to the left of the ferry terminal.

Stage II: Together we walked from home to the train station, bought tickets, caught the train to Circular Quay and went to Wharf 3. This time I waved my father off on the ferry and cheerfully went to work, knowing that Marko would be waiting for him at the other end. Eight hours later I met him as he came off the ferry and we made our way home together.

Stage III: Together we walked from home to the train station, where I bought him a ticket and asked the stationmaster if I could see my father off from the platform. I ecstatically walked back home.

Stage IV: For the final, successful journey, Dad left the house on his own with a piece of paper in his pocket on which was written: "When you get to the station, ask for a Senior Citizen's Day Tripper, which will cost $2.50. Go to platform 7. Check the indicator board to make sure the train is going to Circular Quay. Get off the train at Circular Quay. Walk out of the platform on the side of the harbour. Go to Wharf 3. Your Day Tripper ticket will allow you to catch the ferry to Manly. When you get to Manly, Marko will be waiting for you at the bus-stop to the left."

Essential to progress is the acknowledgement and celebration of every step forward. When a baby is learning to walk, the faintest hint of progress excites us. We encourage, clap, squeal and make a big fuss over every milestone. We give constant positive reinforcement. Why don't we celebrate achievements in the same way when we're adults? Our need for encouragement, acknowledgement and celebration doesn't diminish as we age. Pleasurable rewards actually help to consolidate changes in our brains that occur when we learn a new skill because pleasure and learning share several of the same neurotransmitters (chemical messengers).

Seesaw

We don't stop playing because we grow old. We grow old because we stop playing.
George Bernard Shaw

The ageing brain behaves like a seesaw. As certain abilities go down, other abilities go up, thereby maintaining—if not improving—our overall ability to function and relate to the world. What seems to receive the biggest blow is our perception of ourselves. We live in a culture that keeps meticulous score of our misses but overlooks most of our hits. I mentioned this to my father. When I related to friends the academic discussions I had with Dad around the kitchen table, they were amazed that Dad was au fait with it all. Medical debates between Mum and me were commonplace in our home, and Dad must have absorbed a lot of jargon just by being around us.

"We're a critical bunch," I began. "We're promptly aware of our slightest shortcomings but slow to recognise when we excel at things. There's no denying we get slower at processing information and sometimes it takes longer to learn certain new skills, but once we've learnt those new skills we're better at applying them in the real world. Yet we take the latter for granted and overemphasise the former. Studies involving pilots, air traffic controllers, bank managers, chess players and bridge players show that when it's a question of speed, those in their twenties perform better in their roles than those in their fifties. But when it comes to extrapolating data, making decisions, recognising patterns and integrating multiple layers of information, those aged fifty-plus are more proficient than their younger counterparts.

"Part of the explanation for this is that as we practise something, we develop thicker myelin sheaths around the nerve and brain cell axons that carry out that activity. Axons are the long cords that transmit electrical signals from one nerve cell to another. Wrapped around most axons is a layer of white, fatty tissue called myelin; this is the white matter of the brain. Myelin insulates the axon and increases the speed of the impulse. The more often we fire electrical signals down an axon, the thicker its myelin sheath becomes. The thicker the myelin sheath, the more effectively brain cells communicate with one another and this translates into being more skilled at something."

"You can't tell me memory skills get better with age," Dad accurately objected.

"I'm not telling you that. Memory for names and contexts does diminish. But our capacity to extract information from our immediate environment and compare it with what we already know gets better. Which would you rather have—speed and memory or discernment and logic? A completely valid way of looking at the brain would be to say we need to think faster and remember things better in youth, to compensate for *not yet having* the superior vocabulary and spatial skills we acquire when we've been around for more than half a century. As we age, we use *more* of our brains, not less. We grasp the bigger picture and understand the essence of an argument more quickly in our fifties than in our twenties. But all we notice is that we can't remember if we turned off the stove before leaving the house."

"You seem to forget that I'm almost 80 years old, not 50."

"The principle is the same: shift your focus from what you *can't* do to what you *can* do. Mastery in one area spills into other areas because it increases confidence to try new things. Slowly you'll start to see that you're capable of much more than you give yourself credit for."

My father was dubious. "But I know my brain has lost a lot of its functions—and I'll never regain them."

"Not so. Brain scans have confirmed that even after losing major functions, say due to a stroke, the brain can reorganise itself to find new ways of performing the lost functions, providing we give it the appropriate input. Standard rehab isn't enough; it's too little effort for too short a time. To see change you need to practise and practise and practise, and gradually the brain rearranges its structure and reallocates or borrows territory from another function—without compromising that function— to replace the territory that was damaged by the stroke. I know you haven't had a stroke but the nature of the damage doesn't matter. It's the response to the damage that determines whether or not you regain the function.

"If we put demands on the brain, it'll find ways to fill the order because that's what the brain is designed to do. It thrives on solving problems. Your brain is just waiting for you to give it a challenge to demonstrate its ingenuity. The problem is that we live in a quick-fix society and people give up too soon. But *I* don't give up. You and I are going to systematically work on the things you find difficult to bring them up to speed."

Dad gave me a weary look. "Great. I can't wait."

Focus

*It is during our darkest moments that we must focus
to see the light.*
Aristotle Onassis

I love trampolines. I've also sustained more injuries on trampolines than anyone I know. But it doesn't deter me from having a jump whenever I come across one. A few years ago I was at Brisbane's night markets, where some huge trampolines had been set up for children. I watched as 10 year-olds were strapped into harnesses, so they could jump to great heights without fear of flying off into the bushes. I had to have a turn.

The young man supervising the operation gave me a bemused look but took my money and connected me to the thick, elasticised ropes. I began bouncing with great gusto. True to form, I landed nowhere near the centre of the trampoline—I was always just short of falling off the edges, but the ropes were there to rescue me every time.

When my time was up, the affable young man couldn't hold back. "That was very impressive," he grinned. "I've never seen anyone miss the bull's-eye so consistently. It's like you had a magnet drawing you off to the sides. But I figured out your problem. You were always *looking* off to the sides. You never once looked down at the middle of the trampoline. If you look there, that's where you'll land."

I thought about his advice for a minute. The crowds had thinned and the temptation was too great. "OK, I'll give it another go."

Back in the harness, I propelled myself into the air and fixed my eyes on the centre of the trampoline. I couldn't believe it—I landed where I looked! I kept my focus on the target and got the same result, over and over again. I was a trampolining legend!

When I glanced over to the side, sure enough, that's where I headed. I looked back to the centre and I was back on track. I laughed for the entire "ride" and then thanked my young wizard for the life lesson: what we focus on is where we end up.

I began to apply this lesson to my father.

I *never* mentioned his forgetfulness. Whenever he felt he'd made a mistake, I casually commented that mistakes were stepping stones and that "failure" was feedback. When he reminded me one morning that we needed to pick up the dry-cleaning, I was ecstatic! Where did that come from? I didn't care. I thanked him repeatedly for remembering and kept referring back to the episode as evidence that his neurons were working just fine.

When he helped me peel potatoes, I told him he was a good kitchen hand. When we tidied his sock drawer together, I told him he was good at sorting. When we went through all his shoes and bundled up a bagful for St Vincent de Paul's, I told him he was methodical and decisive. When he returned home after a successful shopping expedition, I told him he was competent and capable. When he helped me carry the bags, I told him he was strong. When he brought the correct documents to appointments, I told him he was organised (even though I'd put the papers in his bag). When he hung out the washing, I told him he was efficient. When he took out the rubbish, I told him he was indispensable. When we walked to the post office, I told him he was fit and sprightly. When he was out of the house and I was left on my own, I collapsed in exhaustion.

All the positive reinforcement was an example of **commanding the crew**—programming his subconscious mind to become what I was telling him he already was.

I began colour-coding the days of the week, hoping it might be a subconscious trigger for remembering what day it was. On Mondays I always used red plates with red serviettes and moved the red vase to the kitchen windowsill. Tuesdays featured orange dishes, an orange tablecloth and orange vase. Wednesdays were yellow, Thursdays green, Fridays blue, Saturdays brown and Sundays white. Where did I find all the different coloured crockery, you might ask? My mother had been a shopaholic and a hoarder. I'd always thought this was a lethal combination but in the current circumstances I was grateful for it.

For a few weeks I never asked Dad what day it was but I mentioned it whenever I was handing him an item of the corresponding colour. I also established routines he could link to specific days of the week. On Sundays I encouraged him to continue going to church. On Monday and Thursday afternoons we went swimming together. On Tuesdays he went to Manly to meet his friend Marko. On Wednesdays I took him to Men's Shed. On Thursday mornings we did Meals on Wheels. Fridays were excursion days, with either me or his delightful 80 year-old friend, Sabine. On Saturdays we picked a section of the house to tidy.

Four weeks after these changes, I asked him what day it was. He hesitated for a moment then answered, "I think it's Monday, isn't it?"

"Yes!" I blinked back tears.

Whenever Dad noticed problems with his memory, he became very distressed. It broke my heart to watch his frustration over forgetting where he'd placed something. It meant so much to see even the slightest improvement. We waltzed to his favourite CD that evening to celebrate.

Revelation

The world is not dangerous because of those who do harm but because of those who look at it without doing anything.
Albert Einstein

During one of our Saturday tidy-ups, Dad and I tackled the fridges—yes, fridges plural. My parents had two full-sized fridges in one undersized kitchen. Not a regular fridge and bar fridge, but two heavy-duty, heavily stocked fridges. I had been longing to purge them for months.

Food plays a critical role in Serbian culture. Feeding me was my mother and grandmother's language of love. Feeding guests at any time of day or night was the bare minimum of hospitality. It was sacrilegious to waste food. Discarding something, even if it was a month past its expiry date, was profligate. So it came as no surprise to find sundried tomatoes due for consumption in 1998 and pickled cucumbers dating back to 1981. The identity of some items was indiscernible.

"What's this?" I asked my father, holding up an unlabelled jar of a creamy-white, semi-hard, odourless substance. "It looks like lard."

"It *is* lard," Dad replied.

"What did you use it for? I don't remember Mum cooking with it."

"Your mother was using it to fatten you up." The colour instantly drained from my face. "Since she thought you didn't eat enough," my father continued, "and your favourite part of chicken was the breast, she used to inject the chicken breast with lard before serving it to you."

I had to sit down for fear of passing out.

Part III
Science Meets Stubbornness

Alice said nothing: she had never been so much contradicted in her life before, and she felt that she was losing her temper.

From *Alice In Wonderland* by Lewis Carroll

Charmed Life

To sit in the shade on a fine day and look upon verdure is the most perfect refreshment.
From *Mansfield Park* by Jane Austen

Prior to my mother's diagnosis, I'd lived a charmed life. Dad was right—I had been responsible for no-one other than myself. I was a happy, serial monogamist. I lived on the top floor of a new, CBD apartment block in balmy Brisbane. My front garden was a 16-hectare, subtropical parkland of lush rainforest ferns, meandering duck-filled lakes and vibrantly coloured, sculpted flowerbeds—the largest urban subtropical garden in the world.

My daily meditation was strolling to work over misty board-walks and cascading waterways. (OK, sometimes it was power walking and sometimes my own mental noise obscured the friendly ibises that gracefully crossed my path.) I never failed to stop at the water-lilies, entranced as I was by their fresh, gorgeous, gelato colours: lemon, mixed berry, blood orange and of course, pristine vanilla. They were delicate yet confident and radiantly beautiful. Their smooth, elegant petals unfurled to smile at the morning sun and gently wrapped around their stamens when it was time for sleep. They were a daily gift to my soul.

On the weekend, I'd sit on my balcony and gaze over the web of pathways and young macadamia nut trees to the dramatic water wall and living floral mural. On warm summer evenings, friends and I would take a picnic to the open air amphitheatre and watch the Queensland Shakespeare Ensemble perform one of the Bard's comedies.

My apartment was light, breezy and deliberately uncluttered. The second bedroom was my office and library, with books arranged by subject and subcategorised alphabetically by author.

One bookshelf for fiction, the other for nonfiction. I had colour coordinated sock drawers.

My friends strongly advised me against having children.

I loved work and enjoyed the company of my workmates at every stage of my career. Exactly a year before my mother had rung with her devastating news, I'd begun a transition from clinical practice to conference platform because I believed that *education* was more powerful than *medication*. Given that eight out of 10 visits to the GP were due to lifestyle factors, I'd become evangelical about people taking responsibility for their own health. Medical science was increasingly recognising how our day-to-day choices have a profound impact on our energy, vitality and immunity to disease.

Every fourth Saturday I flew to Sydney to do a day's work at a medical practice so I'd have a tax-deductible excuse to subscribe to the Sydney Theatre Company and to catch up with friends and, of course, to see my parents. I'd moved from Sydney to Brisbane on Valentine's Day 2004 because my boyfriend at the time lived in Brisbane; it was easier for me to transport my life north than for him to relocate south. The relationship ended after three years but we remain good friends. A few years later I started dating a Sydney man — the aforementioned Dan — so once again I was in a long-distance relationship. This time it was to remain long-distance because I felt very settled in Brisbane, the price of real estate was far less crippling than in Sydney and I loved the climate. Likewise, Dan was established in Sydney and had two young children who could not be uprooted. We were both very comfortable with the arrangement.

BEEP

I find television very educational. Every time someone switches it on, I go into another room and read a good book.
Groucho Marx

Grief can strike at the most unpredictable and inconvenient times.

I'd bought tickets for Dad and his friend, Sabine, to see the Chinese classical dance company, Shen Yun, perform at Luna Park. Dozens of dazzling, exotic, acrobatic dancers graced a spectacular stage to deliver inspiring stories from history and mythology—such was the description on the website. I knew they'd both love it, and they did. It had been decades since my father had been to Luna Park and he wondered if we could ride the huge ferris wheel. Of course we could!

I delivered the two of them to the performance and then sought a quiet place in a park so I could catch up on reading and paperwork. I was looking forward to three uninterrupted hours of solitude. On the way out, I stopped to buy tickets for the ferris wheel, so we could all ride it after the show. As I walked through Luna Park's famed, open-mouthed entrance, I was suddenly overcome by sadness. Unable to articulate what was happening, I broke out in great, child-like sobs. I ran to find a secluded patch of grass and buried my head in my hands. I sobbed for a long time, the kind of sobs that stay written on your face for hours: the red creases, the puffy eyes, the swollen, anaesthetised lips.

I seldom allowed myself to conceive of the enormity of my father's loss and the deep desolation he must be feeling. He'd always had an ingenuous innocence and vulnerability about him, and now it was more pronounced than ever. There had always been a tinge of sadness about him as well, as though he was constantly standing half in shadow. I didn't understand it but every so often I felt it.

So much for my paperwork—I wrapped my scarf around my head for camouflage and returned to collect Sabine and my father.

Shen Yun and Luna Park were part of the Big Environmental Enrichment Plan (BEEP) I'd drawn up for Dad. Our brain cells produce different proteins when we find ourselves in a **stimulating environment** versus a monotonous environment. This happens within just a few hours of a change in our surroundings. After a year of environmental enrichment in which social, physical and mental activity is stimulated, not only do we increase the number of brain cells we have, we increase the number of connections between them by 200–300 per cent! And the number of connections between brain cells (known as synapses) correlates directly with our mental performance: the more synapses, the better our brains operate. **Education** alone increases brain volume, blood supply, cell branches and cell connections.

Research demonstrates that mice placed in big enclosures with lots of other mice to play with, and given a diverse range of games, toys and labyrinths to amuse themselves with, outperform lonely mice in boring cages in every way they're tested. Rats that have a range of tunnels, treadmills and mazes to explore have heavier brains with better blood supplies and more neurotransmitters compared to rats that are not given as much stimulation. In fact, animals of any species raised in stimulating environments learn better than their counterparts in impoverished environments. It all relates to the three key ingredients of a healthy brain: social, physical and mental stimulation.

If a kitten's eye is sewn shut at birth and then re-opened two months later, the kitten becomes blind in that eye—without visual stimulation, the part of the brain responsible for processing information from that eye fails to develop. The brain is literally shaped by its environment. Humans are the same. The more our senses are stimulated, the more invigorating it is for our brains.

This was the rationale of BEEP. Dad and I went on excursions to the beach, galleries and museums. We watched foreign films with subtitles. We went to literary lunches. We sampled Korean, Tibetan and Cambodian food. We took ourselves to Canberra to watch Dan perform in a musical. We went to Homebush Olympic Pool twice a week; my father to enjoy the spas and water jets and me to enjoy my rhythmic laps. I encouraged him to walk barefoot over different surfaces: grass, sand, moss, pebbles, flowing water and squishy mud.

"Focus on your feet and really enjoy the experience," I encouraged.

"I'm happy to do what you tell me for once. But why?"

"When you **walk barefoot**, especially over uneven surfaces, your brain receives diverse input from the soles of your feet, which leads to better balance. It's another myth that as we age we inevitably get frail and unsteady on our feet. We start to feel unsure on our feet because we haven't been feeling our way as we walk—our feet have been cocooned in shoes for 70-plus years.

"And don't look down," I instructed. "Rely on your feet to send you signals about how to maintain your balance. Stimulating the soles of your feet also stimulates your soul in here." I touched his chest. "And it changes the architecture of your brain."

"I'm too old for changes in my brain."

"I have news for you. Your brain is *constantly* changing throughout your entire life—whether you want it to or not—and *you're* driving that change by what you do, think and experience. So you may as well do, think and experience things that drive positive change, rather than negative change." I paused before giving him a metaphor he'd relate to: "Your brain is continually rewiring itself and you're the electrician."

Beans

If I believe I cannot do something, it makes me incapable of doing it. But when I believe I can, then I acquire the ability to do it, even if I didn't have it in the beginning.
Mahatma Gandhi

It was Good Friday and my father was drinking black coffee. This was unusual because he always had milk in his coffee. We weren't out of milk but I asked anyway.

"No, we have milk," he replied. "Have you forgotten that it's Good Friday? We're not allowed to consume any animal products, dairy included."

It was a long time since I'd spent Good Friday with my parents, and I had no recollection of it being a day of fasting.

"You have to cook beans today. Your mother always cooked bean stew on Good Friday," he insisted.

"I would be happy to cook beans today, but being Good Friday no supermarkets or stores will be open and we don't have any beans at home." We had recently cleaned out the kitchen cupboards and there were no beans.

"I'll show you," he replied and took me into the laundry. Pushing aside a row of cleaning rags, he revealed six packets of borlotti beans. Of course—the laundry. Why hadn't I thought of looking there?

"That's great but I still can't cook bean stew today because we don't have the other ingredients: no tomatoes or other vegies, not even an onion. I was planning to have last night's vegetarian frittata tonight, but that won't work unless we pick the egg and cheese out of it."

"In that talk of yours I attended a few weeks ago," Dad countered, "you said to cut the word 'can't' out of our vocabulary because the brain is very sensitive and responsive to language. Whenever we say 'can't', it's like choking the brain, putting it in a straitjacket or giving it a restraining order. Swap 'can't' for 'how' and you'll get your brain working for you to find solutions. So don't tell me you can't make beans on Good Friday."

I had to leave the room to stop from screaming. How could he remember exactly what I'd said in a talk more than two weeks ago but he couldn't remember what I'd said five minutes ago? It made no sense whatsoever. The unpredictability of his memory was maddening.

After a few deep breaths, I pondered *how* I was going to make a tasty bean stew without a recipe and ingredients. Much as I was loath to admit it, Dad was right. Everything we say to ourselves has the effect of giving our brains an instruction. If I say, "I can't make bean stew," I dampen my brain cell activity. If I ask, "How can I make bean stew?" I'm instructing my brain cells to come up with a creative solution.

"I've asked myself how I'm going to make bean stew, so let's sit with it for a while and see what bright ideas come up for either of us."

"That's a better attitude." My father didn't even look up from his Sudoku.

Come five o'clock, there were no bright ideas, but I had to tackle the beans regardless. The packet said to cook them in plenty of water for two hours; surely I'd come up with something by then. Plenty of water was an understatement. No sooner had I turned my back, they'd soaked up all the water and started sticking to the saucepan. Meanwhile I was searching the kitchen *and* the laundry in the hope that something would occur to me.

I scrounged up half a carrot, half a celery stick, three cloves of garlic, half a cup of capers, three fresh chillies from the garden, a jar of paprika and a tin of pumpkin soup. I threw all of it—yes, all of it, including the jar of paprika—into a non-stick frying pan. The bulk paprika wasn't intentional but the lid fell off and most of the contents of the jar went in. This was actually a good thing because my father claimed he didn't eat pumpkin but he did enjoy spicy food. So I disguised the taste of the pumpkin by burning his tongue off. Unpalatable and unlikely as it sounds, when I added the beans—which were tasteless on their own—it looked like a bean stew, with no hint of pumpkin because the paprika had dyed everything red. As for the taste, well, I'll never know. Between the chillies and the paprika, neither of us had any taste buds left.

Commands

If you think you can do a thing or think you can't do a thing, you're right.
Henry Ford

Even though Dad was quick to admonish me for saying "can't", he found it entirely acceptable as part of his own vocabulary. So I told him the following story.

"Once upon a time, there was a captain of a boat with a very loyal and competent crew. They were the most faithful crew you could ever imagine—anything the captain ordered, the crew carried out. They never questioned the captain's judgement and they never spoke back to him. The captain was the unilateral decision maker, and the crew worked around the clock carrying out the captain's orders.

"The captain didn't know how his crew accomplished everything because all he had to do was announce his orders. If he needed information, the crew would find it and present it to him. If he needed a job done, they'd do it exactly as asked. Yet despite this seemingly ideal situation, where his every command was followed to the letter, the captain was running into trouble.

"The crew couldn't cope with wishy-washy orders. They couldn't think for themselves, so they needed very precise and detailed instructions about what the captain wanted. To make matters worse, the crew never asked the captain to clarify an order. If they weren't sure what the captain wanted, they'd follow a well-trodden path of least resistance, which often led to poor results. This frustrated the captain because he didn't realise the problem was his imprecise orders.

"Another reason the captain ran into trouble was that he didn't know the crew eavesdropped on his every conversation. They interpreted everything he said as a command, whether he intended it as one or not. When the captain said to himself, 'This is going to be a bad day', the crew interpreted it as, '*Give* me a bad day'. When he said, 'This situation is hopeless' or 'I can't do this', the crew stopped working altogether.

"The captain was also unaware that the crew had no sense of humour; they took everything literally. When the captain joked about having a bad memory, the crew took it as meaning it was unimportant to remember something. So they failed to record the information and it turned the joke into a self-fulfilling truth." I paused for emphasis.

"I presume there's a point to this story?" my father asked.

"The captain represents your conscious mind and the crew represent your subconscious mind. Everything you say, either aloud or to yourself, is an instruction to your subconscious mind. And it operates exactly like the crew operate—to the letter. Every time you say to me, 'I'm too old for this' or 'I'm always losing things' or 'I can't learn new things at my age,' you're programming yourself for failure. You need to consciously **command your crew. Change your language and you change your life.** Not only does what we say change our perspective and attitude, it changes our brains. Our self-talk has a physical impact on our brain cells: it can either fire them up or dampen them down. So watch your language!"

"But I *do* have a bad memory. It's a fact," Dad contended.

"No, it's not a fact. You've extrapolated that having occasional memory lapses means you have a bad memory overall. Too often, after a slip-up, we magnify the error and believe it's a sign that our overall functioning is deteriorating. Stop making negative generalisations about yourself. Yes, you sometimes forget things but that doesn't mean you have a bad memory. It means you aren't *using* your memory. You don't have a memory problem so much as you have a communication problem between your captain and crew, between your conscious and subconscious mind. You've allowed your memory to go into retirement by labelling yourself as having a bad memory and by telling yourself you're old and have permission to be forgetful. Get it out of retirement by telling your memory it has to keep working. Every time you want to remember something, say to yourself, 'This is important and I can and will remember it'."

"It's not normal to talk to yourself like that," he objected. "It feels forced and unnatural."

"It only feels unnatural because you're in the habit of speaking negatively about yourself. It's just a habit. Break it by becoming conscious of it."

"And how do you propose I do that?"

I went to the cupboard and brought to the table two large glass jars.

"This is *your* Can-Do Jar and this is *my* Can-Do Jar. Every time you or I say the word 'can't' or any of its cousins, such as 'impossible', 'too hard' or 'I'm too old', we have to put a gold coin in our jar. If your jar gets full, I get to spend the money. If my jar gets full, *you* get to spend the money."

"That's not fair. I'm older than you and my habits are much more ingrained than yours. Besides, I have a lot more to complain about than you."

"That's two gold coins in your jar already!"

"What?"

"You just put yourself down twice. Pay up."

"Hang on, let's get clear on the rules. You're saying it will cost a gold coin every time one of us complains about something? Even one teensy-weensy negative thing?"

"Yes."

"That's unrealistic."

"No, it just takes practice. Practise minding your language and catching your thoughts. Talk and think about what's going *right* for you, not about what's going wrong. It will be challenging to start with, but if you persevere, being positive will become a habit, just as being negative is a habit."

He shook his head. "My one advantage is that you talk a lot more than I do, so you're bound to complain about something sooner or later."

Curiosity

The important thing is not to stop questioning ...
Never lose a holy curiosity.
Albert Einstein

Nature abhors a vacuum. When we remove the word "can't" from our vocabulary, it leaves a void that wants to be filled — and the perfect fit is "how". The word "how" has the opposite effect on the brain to the word "can't". **If we replace "can't" with "how", we instantly change our mindset from one of despair to one of repair.**

Asking solution-focused "how" questions, such as, "How can I work with this situation, even though it wasn't part of my plans?" gives the subconscious mind a directive to find the answer. Our brains are wired in such a way that we see whatever it is we're looking for. Our eyes merely convert light into electrical impulses, which are sent to the brain for interpretation. But our interpretation of what we see is highly subjective and influenced by our beliefs and expectations. If we expect an answer will be forthcoming when we ask a question, then something we see, hear or experience will guide us to that answer, or will act as a trigger for the answer to come to mind.

Have you ever noticed that when you buy a new car or even consider buying a certain model, suddenly it seems to be the most common car on the road? Or when you've just had a relationship break-up, everywhere you look, you see reminders of what could have been, should have been and would have been? Such is the subjective nature of our perceptions, and it works in the same way when we live with a can-do attitude versus a complaining attitude. The more we complain, the more we find to complain about. The more we ask "How?" the more we find answers coming our way. All that's required is persistence and a bit of patience.

One thing working against this is our culture of instant gratification. We are often too impatient for answers, throwing our hands up in despair if the solution isn't immediately evident. Yet consistently asking ourselves (or others), "How can this be achieved?" instead of "This can't be done", or "How can I communicate more effectively with this person?" instead of "I can't get through to this person", places us on alert for solutions. We then subconsciously scan our environment for clues to steer us in the right direction. When asking "how" questions becomes a habit, we experience "fortunate coincidences" and sense that things are falling into place—what we're doing is **commanding our crew** to seek out the answers we need.

Asking "How?" also switches on our innate curiosity, a vastly underrated faculty. Einstein said, "Curiosity has its own reason for existence", and neuroscientists have discovered what that reason is: **curiosity keeps our brains sharp, active and alive**.

Curiosity drives us to learn, explore and live life to the full, till the day we die. It induces our brains to get creative and find solutions. Being curious makes us pay attention, thereby aiding learning and memory. It's an active state that strengthens problem-solving skills—asking questions trains our minds to invent and innovate.

Curiosity has many virtues. Curious people are more resilient, observant and resourceful. They are more likely to ask "Why?" or "Where to from here?" They seek reasons and answers, rather than pass judgement or feel defeated. Curiosity allows us to live in a world of adventure and possibility. It boosts our brains because it creates a perceptual filter for useful information in our environment. Curiosity is a powerful motivating factor towards mastery, expertise and scientific discovery.

Importantly, curiosity stops us from blind acceptance and from rushing into things—in this way, curiosity equates to power. It protects us from falling prey to advertising and fraudulent offers.

Curiosity in others signals interest and attraction; ongoing curiosity helps sustain romance. Curiosity is an ingredient of compassion and understanding. What drove this person to behave in this way? What made them choose one course of action over another? What lies behind their decision?

Curiosity is a guide to our strengths and passions. If we're curious about a subject, we become more knowledgeable about it, develop related skills and acquire a level of expertise in proportion to our curiosity. Curiosity leads us to engage in other brain-boosting pursuits, such as further education, new hobbies and meeting new people.

Curiosity increases activity in the brain's hippocampus and enhances the recall of answers to trivia questions. Curiosity also activates our imaginations—and imagination is a powerful brain booster in its own right.

With respect to my father, what I valued most about cultivating curiosity was that it served as an antidote to my judgements. **Curious not critical** became my sanity-saving mantra. To stop myself from labelling something he did or didn't do as a sign of laziness, apathy, inertia, inconsideration or unfairness, I'd ask myself, "Why might he have no motivation to participate? What could be going on for him right now? What is he trying to communicate? What might he be feeling? What makes him think that way?"

Sometimes I asked him the question, but more often merely posing it to myself reminded me that whatever he was doing made perfect sense to him—we're all doing the best we can, based on our resources and accumulated life experiences.

Despite my best intentions, I confess that I nonetheless occasionally blurted out, "Where in the rule book of life does it say you're allowed to abdicate responsibility for yourself and fob it off on me?" But on the whole, I maintained my composure.

Dad seemed to have lost most of his own curiosity long ago. How could I help him rekindle it? A motivated individual will make a conscious effort to be more curious once they become aware of the power of curiosity. Other steps include:

- Get into the habit of asking questions—any question about anything.
- Question your beliefs and assumptions if they aren't useful or uplifting.
- Become interested in what motivates others.
- If someone does something that upsets, frustrates or angers you, think about how they may have justified their actions.
- Become more observant. Take time to notice life's details.
- Read about a wide range of subjects, unrelated to your work.
- Your reading doesn't have to be of thick texts; short articles can be very effective in stimulating curiosity.
- Regularly speak to people you don't know.

When I first suggested to my father that he replace "can't" with "how", he played along facetiously. "How do I do that?" he asked, dozens of times every day. In some cases, I'd show him; other times I would reflect the question back to him. When he asked me what he should wear, I'd reply, "What do you think would be the most appropriate thing to wear?" When he asked how I expected him to use the washing machine, when he had no idea what to do, I answered, "Look at the buttons on the front panel. If you had to guess which buttons to press and which dials to turn to get it going, what would you do?" I needed to repeat the instructions every week but it didn't matter. The point was for him to practise curiosity, so that eventually curiosity would become a life-enhancing habit. (If you're concerned that curiosity killed the cat, the original proverb is actually "care killed the cat", where care means sorrow or worry. Besides, if curiosity killed the cat, "satisfaction brought it back".)

Connection

No man is an island, entire of itself; every man is a piece of the continent, a part of the main.
John Donne

The brain is a social beast. It loves company, thriving on connection and social interaction with others.

There is plenty of evidence for this. A recent English study found that people in their 50s and 60s who socialised more frequently had better cognitive skills than people who kept to themselves. Researchers at the University of Miami recorded that people living in apartments with balconies facing the street, which encouraged conversations with neighbours and passers-by, had better mental functioning than people whose residences were more isolated. A US study of 3000 elderly people in 1999 found those with no social contacts had almost twice the risk of developing cognitive problems as those who had five or more social contacts. Also in the 1990s, Swedish researchers tracked more than 1200 elderly people for three years and found that those who reported satisfying social contacts were 40 per cent less likely to develop dementia than those with few or unsatisfying relationships. Similarly, a rich social network and meaningful relationships reduce the risk of depression, and depression itself is a risk factor for dementia and has been linked to shrinkage of the hippocampus. Conversely, older people who reported feeling lonely were twice as likely to develop Alzheimer's Disease as their more socially connected and communicative counterparts. Living with someone into old age also cuts our risk of Alzheimer's by more than 60 per cent.

Even lab rats allowed to play with human children are better learners than lab rats left alone in their cage.

Dad needed to **connect with fellow travellers**. My first target was Men's Shed.

Men's Shed is a uniquely Australian concept, where men get together in a shed for one or two days each week to do what many men like to do: build boats, restore furniture, fix toys, tinker with tools and talk about sport—or even share life experiences. Sometimes they make things for charities or repair bikes for family and friends. There are Men's Sheds all around the country, providing supportive and relaxed environments for men to do as much or as little work as they choose, or simply lend a hand or a listening ear.

I decided this would be absolutely perfect for my father. I googled our nearest Shed and found to my great delight that it was only a 10-minute drive away—just close enough for Dad to drive himself when he became confident about how to get there. It was meant to be! I casually began bringing up Men's Shed in conversation, so he'd gradually warm to the idea. Each time, I was met with unqualified resistance. He had no inclination, no interest and no reason to go. On the contrary, I suggested, it would do his mind and mood a world of good. "No," he stated. I knew this was only a manifestation of his grief and fear of the unknown, so I cheerfully kept at it. On the evening before the first visit, I nonchalantly reminded him that we had a fun outing planned for the next day.

"No!"

I was so excited I could hardly sleep, just like a child on Christmas Eve. Men's Shed was a gift to my father and me. It ticked all the boxes: it provided a new and interesting environment (**docking the boat in stimulating surroundings**), an opportunity to learn new skills (**learning new ropes**), and a support network and social stimulation (**connecting with fellow travellers**). It offered the ultimate in brain boosting for Dad and a free day for *me* (caring for the carer). I started fantasising about all the things I could do with six uninterrupted hours!

This particular Men's Shed operated from 10 am to 3 or 4 pm on Wednesdays and Saturdays. We'd start with Wednesdays and then add Saturdays as he became more familiar with the group and more comfortable attending. I woke up before the alarm and happily went about preparing my father's lunch: homemade chicken caesar salad (minus the croutons) and a small banana. I'd bought a yellow lunchbox because it was Wednesday. To a yellow plastic bag I added plastic cutlery, a yellow serviette, a toothpick and his denture glue—and I sighed in contentment. I went to wake Dad.

"But I don't want to go to Men's Shed!" he objected.

"Let's just go and take a look. I promised the nice man who runs it that we'd pay a visit today. If you don't like it, we'll come home. You're under no obligation to stay if you hate it. But you can't reject it outright without first seeing what it's about. When I was a child you always told me to give something a fair go before I wrote it off."

"I'm old enough to know what I will and won't like." He remained unmoved.

"Please? Just this once? Just to get me off your case?" He sighed.

"OK, now here's your lunch …"

"I won't need it," he interrupted. "I won't be staying that long."

"Well, just in case. I like to be prepared."

He complained during the entire drive. I decided not to broach the subject of him driving himself on future visits. On arrival, the very friendly and welcoming Steve greeted us.

"Hello! You must be Helena. And this is your dad, Ilija? I've been practising the pronunciation. Did I get it right?"

"Yes, perfect." I couldn't help feeling at ease in Steve's presence, and I smiled at Dad. He averted his eyes.

"Come in and take a look around," Steve invited. I all but skipped in.

Steve showed us around and started talking about their latest project: a cubby house for a charity raffle. It looked fabulous.

"I can't do this," my father said. "I've never made a cubby house before."

"Neither have I," reassured Steve. "We're all learning on the job—that's what it's all about. We'll get you doing things you can manage."

My father pulled me aside. "I don't want to be here."

"I know this is all new and unfamiliar and potentially unnerving for you," I said, "but that's not a bad thing. Everything feels awkward the first time we try it. It will do your brain a world of good being in a different environment with different people doing different things. It's as powerful as any of the medications you're taking. Just give it a go for one hour, and if you're unhappy ring me and I'll come and pick you up. Just one hour— that's all I ask."

I left Dad in Steve's kind and capable hands, asking him to ring me in an hour, just to let me know how things were going.

I collapsed in a heap when I arrived home. I just lay there for what seemed a very long time. Then I sent an SMS to my friend, Marina: "I know what it was like for you on Simon's first day of school. I take my hat off to you." The minute I pressed Send, I was overcome by guilt and sadness. I felt as though I'd betrayed Dad by comparing him to a child. My internal dialogue about Dad was as important as what I said to him. What mattered most was that he felt accepted as a worthwhile human being, who had something left to contribute—but I was treating him like an uncooperative child. I burst into tears.

I jumped when the phone rang. Please, please, let my father want to stay …

"Hi, it's Steve. Your father's totally absorbed in helping with the cubby house. Don't you dare come and disturb him."

"Oh, thank you, thank you so much!" I danced around the living room. At one o'clock the phone rang again. It was my father.

"You have to come and pick me up straight away!"

"Why? What's wrong?"

"Everyone's sitting down to lunch and I don't have anything."

"Yes, you do. Your lunchbox is on the top shelf of the fridge. Ask Steve and he'll show you."

"So when will you come and pick me up?"

"At three o'clock."

"That's too late."

"No, it's not. Everyone else will be staying well past three."

"Come at two o'clock."

"Two-thirty."

"Promise?"

"Yes."

I was getting a headache and my neck was feeling tight—I could really do with a massage. Instead I did a load of washing.

"So how was it?" I buoyantly ventured when I returned to Men's Shed at exactly two-thirty.

Dad shrugged. At least he didn't say he hated it.

"The more often you go, the more you'll enjoy it," I said.

He remained silent.

Reality Check

Keep your sense of proportion by regularly, preferably daily, visiting the natural world.
Caitlin Matthews

The following Wednesday posed an even greater challenge. I was due in Brisbane to speak at a conference, so I wouldn't be able to drive my father to Men's Shed. If he missed his second week, I was afraid we'd go back to square one—I couldn't bear the thought. I couldn't let my client down by cancelling, but I didn't want to let Dad down either. What to do?

The issue wasn't that I couldn't call on someone to drive my father a mere 10 minutes from home; the issue was that Dad would refuse to go. I needed someone who would be patient, willing and skilled enough to coax him into going—my father's psychiatrist! This wasn't as outrageous as it sounds. Clyde had been a close friend and colleague of my mother's and had told me to call on him any time I needed anything. He was a gentle, softly spoken, 60 year-old man with a hesitant gait and a ready smile.

"Of course I'd be delighted to take your father," Clyde said. "What a great idea. It's just what he needs."

"You may encounter some resistance," I warned, "but please be firm and insist that he goes. Tell him it's as powerful for his brain and wellbeing as his medications. Tell him ..."

"Hey, don't sound so worried," laughed Clyde. "I've known your father for years and I know how to handle him."

"This isn't the man you see in a clinical setting. He can be very defiant."

"I've been doing this for a long time and it won't be the first time I've seen defiance. Trust me."

"OK. I just wanted to warn you. And please remember to take his lunch from the fridge."

My presentation was at midday, and I planned to call Clyde mid-morning to see how he was going. At 9.30 am I received a call from a distressed psychiatrist.

"Your father refuses to go to Men's Shed."

"I warned you."

"What will I do?"

"You're asking *me* what to do?" I held back from reminding him of our previous conversation.

"Don't take no for an answer. You're his doctor. He has to listen to you." I hung up.

Fifteen minutes later I received another call from Clyde. "Can I put your father on the phone?"

I spent the next 10 minutes reiterating everything I'd ever said about Men's Shed, adding, "You can't be rude to Clyde, given that he's come to pick you up. Just go with him for today and we'll talk about this when I get home. Why are you being so difficult? Why would I be organising this for you if it wasn't in your absolute and unequivocal best interests?"

Five minutes later, another call from Clyde. "Your father says he can't go because he has no lunch to take."

"I told both of you that it's on the top shelf of the fridge in the yellow lunchbox in the yellow plastic bag!"

Thirty minutes later, another call. I was ready to explode.

"It's all good with your father. As soon as we arrived, he beamed as everyone greeted him and took him to the cubby house. As for me, I'm going home to have a strong drink and a lie down."

Espionage

No man is useless who has a friend.
Robert Louis Stevenson

My second target for **connecting with fellow travellers** was Probus. This association's name is an amalgamation of "professional" and "business". Probus originated in the United Kingdom in 1965 as a group for retired professional or business people who wanted to keep their minds active, their interests expanding and their circle of friends broadening. It has now spread throughout the world and is open to any retiree seeking fellowship, fun and fulfilment. Two ex-Rotarians started Probus and each club is sponsored by a Rotary Club. Members meet at least once a month to fraternise, hear speakers, plan outings, exchange ideas and enjoy life. There is also an organised excursion each month and a week-long trip each year.

Once again, I googled the nearest club: there was one only five minutes from home—even more promising than Men's Shed. And the meetings only lasted two hours, so it would be an easier sell to Dad. I rang to find out about the program.

"Funerals," replied an effervescent voice.

"Funerals?"

"Yes. We have a speaker coming to discuss funerals. People don't like to think about them, but it's so much easier on the family if we make plans ahead of time. We thought the club could talk about funerals and probably have a few laughs while we were at it."

My father wasn't about to have a few laughs over funeral plans. I wished *both* my parents had been to the meeting six months ago.

"What's on the program for next month?"

"A chiropractor is coming to talk about posture, back care and general mobility."

Perfect. This time I tried a different tack with my father.

"Dad, I need to ask a favour. I need you to go and check out a group called Probus. I've been invited to speak at one of their meetings and I know nothing about them. I need you to do some espionage for me." (OK, so I hadn't actually received an invitation to speak …)

"Why can't *you* go to the meeting?" he asked.

"Because it's only for retirees."

"How long does it go for?"

"Two hours."

"OK, I'll do that for you."

When I came to collect him after the meeting, Dad was engrossed in conversation. I happily waited and took the opportunity to offer my speaking services to the secretary. After discussing suitable topics, he took my business card, and I pencilled a tentative date in my diary. Phew. I'd made an honest woman of myself.

O Brother

The least likely teacher might offer you the most to learn.
Brian Beirne

I was extremely grateful for Marko. Marko was the one friend and fellow traveller that I didn't need to encourage Dad to spend time with. Usually my father caught the train and ferry to meet Marko at Manly (I was thrilled I'd been able to teach him how to get there on his own), but sometimes Marko would make the hour-long drive to our home. On several occasions, Marko told me that my father was like a brother to him. Seeing them laugh together in our backyard reminded me of two best school friends. It warmed my heart.

Marko and Dad had met more than 10 years ago at the local RSL Club, where they were celebrating a mutual friend's birthday. The two men immediately hit it off when they discovered they'd grown up in the same street in Belgrade. They'd even both stolen plums from the same bountiful tree. Their commonality of background was reassuring for Dad; so many things didn't need to be said and Dad liked it that way. Marko was about 10 years younger than my father and had two children and three grandchildren. He was thickset, had a pronounced limp and walked with a cane. I asked my father what had happened to Marko's leg, but he didn't know and didn't like to pry. My mother never liked Marko and I couldn't understand why.

One morning, shortly before Dad was to meet Marko, I found him slipping $100 into his wallet.

"What are you doing with Marko today?" I asked, wondering what would cost $100.

"I don't know. I'm just giving Marko $100, so he can pay for his insurance."

"What insurance?"

"I don't know. Marko just said he needed $100 to pay an insurance bill."

"I see."

I *didn't* see. What insurance bill costs $100? Maybe he was $100 short? It sounded a bit odd, but I didn't want to interfere. It was my father's money and if he wanted to help out a friend, so be it. A fortnight later, I walked in on the same scenario.

"Are you taking Marko out to a fancy lunch today?"

"No, Marko needs $50 to pay for his dry-cleaning."

"I've never seen Marko wear a suit. And he must go to a very expensive dry-cleaner."

"I don't know. I'm not about to pry."

"Is Marko in financial trouble?" I ventured. "A few weeks ago you gave him $100 to pay for his insurance."

"No, I didn't."

"Yes, you did."

"I don't remember doing so."

"*I* remember you doing so."

"If *you* remember that Marko needed $100 for his insurance and *I* don't remember it, then *you* must have given him $100, not me."

I couldn't argue with memory loss.

When Dad had gone, I sat down and thought about it. How often was Marko asking my father for money? My mind ran amok with possibilities and permutations.

Likelihood #1: I'd walked in on the only two times in the history of their friendship that Marko had asked for money. Marko was having a particularly difficult month and was embarrassed to admit it. Serbs are a very proud race; you tell people whatever you need to tell them to save face, and when someone borrows your money, you never ask for it back. Marko had told me he regarded Dad as a brother. Financial problems were something you didn't reveal to people outside the immediate family. Therefore, it was actually a compliment to my father that Marko was asking for money.

Likelihood #2: Marko was my father's genuine friend but viewed him as being financially better off and therefore able to spare some cash from time to time. There was nothing sinister about asking for money. Besides, Marko's wife fed the two men hearty, traditional Yugoslav fare before they went out for the afternoon, and I could view the money as a generous contribution to lunch.

Likelihood #3: Marko was a small-time gambler and had decided to latch onto Dad to support his habit.

Likelihood #4: Marko was a leech, and with my mother out of the way, he was planning to use my father for all he could get.

What should I do? The last thing I wanted was to take away Dad's "best friend". He felt a long-standing bond with the man and very much enjoyed their time together. They were good mates and good mates helped each other out. My father also felt he was doing Marko a service by getting him out of the house once a week. The second last thing I wanted was to remove a key brain booster from my father's life. The third last thing I wanted was to rob myself of a free half day each week.

I did the sums. Assuming the worst—Dad was giving Marko $50–$100 per week—then it was costing $75 per week for my father to get fed and socially stimulated, while I got six to seven hours to myself. It was a no-brainer. I would do nothing. If I paid for a carer or diversional therapist (my father wouldn't hear of it) or if I took him to a day respite centre (he would refuse to go), it would cost me a lot more and it wouldn't come close to giving my father the same emotional and psychological benefits. I went to bed at peace with the status quo.

But I awoke in a cold sweat, having dreamed about:

Likelihood #5: Marko had a bigger plan. He was building up Dad's trust, so that one day he could ask him to sign as guarantor on a loan for a dodgy business his son-in-law or cousin or nephew was about to start. A year later, the business would go bust, and we'd lose the house and all our possessions. I'd happily give away most of the possessions, but losing the house would destroy my father. We'd live miserably ever after. This was ridiculous—but possible. Not the "miserably ever after" part because I simply don't "do" miserable, but I didn't need any more curve balls to deal with.

I resolved to tell my father a story about what could happen if a person signed as guarantor for someone else's loan. The chances of him remembering the story were slim, but perhaps if he ever found himself in the situation, it would trigger something in his brain and he'd be careful or at least ask me for advice. Meanwhile, I would find out as much as I could about Marko and keep a close eye on outgoing cash.

Wonderland

*People from a planet without flowers would think we must be
mad with joy the whole time to have such things about us.*
Iris Murdoch

If you can't beat 'em, bribe 'em.

After seeing the movie *Avatar* in 3D, Dad asked if we could also
see *Alice in Wonderland* in 3D. I immediately saw the opportunity
for some bargaining.

"Yes, of course we can," I said, "on Wednesday afternoon, after I
pick you up from Men's Shed."

"Oh."

He said nothing more until Wednesday morning, when I asked
him to get ready for Men's Shed. "Are we going to see *Alice* this
afternoon?"

"Yes, we are."

"You won't be late picking me up, will you?"

"Definitely not."

Alice in Wonderland wouldn't have been my movie of choice but
it was a small price to pay for a debate-free Wednesday morning.
I was pleasantly surprised and found myself identifying with
Alice's plight. As I watched her fall down the rabbit hole, it was
strangely reminiscent of falling into the unfathomable world of
my father. After the movie, I went so far as to re-read the book.
It was comforting to have someone else (even a character in a
fantasy) echo my thoughts. Like Alice, I had spent the first few

weeks pinching myself because my new situation didn't seem real and I wanted to wake up from the dream.

> *The rabbit hole went straight on like a tunnel for some way* (like my mother's illness), *and then dipped suddenly down* (my mother's rapid decline and ultimate death), *so suddenly that Alice had not a moment to think about stopping herself before she found herself falling down a very deep well.* I had operated on autopilot, creating a makeshift bedroom and workspace for myself, while keeping Dad alive, moving, talking, interacting—the things we take for granted until life knocks the wind out of us.

> *Either the well was very deep, or she fell very slowly, for she had plenty of time as she went down to look about her* (I could see that it would be a full-time job to re-engage my father with life), *and to wonder what was going to happen next.* Every day I wondered what was going to happen next.

> *Down, down, down. Would the fall never come to an end!* (Every time I think I see a pattern in Dad's memory loss and behaviour, he does something that completely baffles me.) *"I wonder how many miles I've fallen by this time?" she said aloud. "I must be getting somewhere near the centre of the earth. Let me see: that would be 4000 miles down, I think—" ... for you see Alice had learnt several things of this sort in her lessons in the schoolroom, and though this was not a very good opportunity for showing off her knowledge, as there was no-one to listen to her, still it was good practice to say it over.* Now that I'd dramatically reduced my workload, there was no-one listening to me, but I needed to put the research into practice like never before. My father

was putting everything I'd ever learnt and spoken about to the test.

What struck me most of all was that in order for Alice to enter Wonderland, in order for her to "get out of that dark hall, and wander about among those beds of bright flowers and those cool fountains", Alice had to make *herself* smaller. *She* had to change to experience what Wonderland had to offer.

SOS

To be upset over what you don't have is to waste what you do have.
Ken Keyes

My childhood home was nothing short of Wonderland.

I've mentioned that my mother was a shopaholic. Not the giggling, retail-as-therapy type, but the hard-core hoard-aholic, who was unable to enjoy a remote tropical island holiday because there weren't enough retail options to keep her entertained. Her favourite sport was bargaining, and she'd play anywhere—from flea markets to David Jones to Armani. Shopping was about the experience, the banter, the game and the competition, as much as the possession at the end of it. Add to that a passion for giving and a war-stricken childhood, and the outcome is diabolical.

A month after my mother died, I sent the following email to all my friends:

"Please place your order for ANY household items and I'll deliver them to your door. I guarantee I'll have whatever you need in whatever size, shape, colour and quantity you require: cups, mugs, cutlery, plates, salad bowls, jars, baking dishes, mixing bowls, wooden spoons, plastic containers, vases, coffee grinders, wine glasses, champagne flutes, tablecloths, towels, bed linen, tissues, wetwipes, washing powder, sunscreen, insect repellent, soap, abrasive cleaning agents, non-abrasive cleaning agents, shampoo, conditioner, hand cream, gloves, hats, caps, large T-shirts, umbrellas, handbags, sunglasses, scarves, accessories, socks, stock cubes, salt, pepper, paprika, YOU NAME IT, I'VE GOT IT, MULTIPLES OF IT, THREE LIFETIMES' SUPPLY OF IT. PLEASE HELP ME."

I had never understood my mother's insatiable need for interminable acquisition. The lounge room floor was a distant memory; the sofa was completely obscured by boxes; and the coffee table was buried under clothing, ornaments, cosmetics and handbags. The room was inaccessible to visitors, and my parents had erected a thick, brown, heavy curtain as a partition between the lounge room and the adjoining TV room.

I particularly resented my mother buying things for *my* home. Underneath my apartment building, I had a storage cage in which I kept all the ornaments, vases, cushions, tablecloths, bowls, wall hangings, pitchers, carry bags, suitcases, etc. that my mother had given me over the years. There was no room for them in my apartment, nor did I want or need the stuff. However, if they weren't on display when my mother came to visit, she would immediately notice and get upset. She didn't understand, "No, thank you." So whenever she visited me in Brisbane, I'd spend half a day transforming my apartment into a Turkish bazaar-cum-museum-cum-homeware store. I covered my walls with her prints and tapestries and made certain there wasn't a square millimetre of exposed surface on any shelf or bench top.

My ultimate fantasy was owning two homes: one for me to live in, and one for me to move into when my parents visited. They'd only know about my second home, the one crammed with their eclectic clutter, and I wouldn't get distressed about all the new things my mother continually bought for me. In my younger years I'd argued with her about bringing me things I'd never use, but she was relentless and it only made for an unhappy relationship. Giving gifts was her language of love. It was her way of communicating how much she cared about me—and she obviously cared a lot. In the end I gave up.

Then, exactly two months after my mother passed away, I read an article in *The Sydney Morning Herald* called "The Collectors". It described hoarding as a debilitating pathological condition that has its roots in early childhood. Neural imaging studies in the US showed that specific parts of the brain were activated in hoarders when they engaged in their addiction, just as other parts of the brain were activated in people with obsessive compulsive disorder. An Australian study had found that growing up in households lacking emotional warmth, and failing to connect with parents, was a possible risk factor for becoming a hoarder. These individuals found comfort in "things" because "things" would not reject them. I thought about my mother's relationship with her own mother and cried.

Pomegranates

Being defeated is often a temporary condition.
Giving up is what makes it permanent.
Marilyn vos Savant

I had no idea that non-stick baking paper had an expiry date; it loses its non-stick properties after sitting in a kitchen drawer for 25 years. I discovered this on the day that Dan, his parents, his brother, his brother's wife and his cousin came to dinner. I thought it would lift my father's morale if the two of us worked on a joint project, so I invited our guests to a mini-banquet.

First thing in the morning I set out to make a choc-macadamia nut-goji berry panforte. The recipe didn't actually include goji berries, but my father had surreptitiously eaten the raisins the previous evening, so I substituted with the next-closest ingredient in the house. Goji berries have a higher antioxidant score than raisins, so my guests were getting a bonus. However when the panforte cooled down, I discovered why goji berries were not in the recipe; after 30 minutes in the oven, they turn into cement pellets that cause serious havoc to dentures. But I digress.

When it was time to peel the baking paper from the panforte, nothing happened. It was inseparable from the cake. After two broken fingernails I eventually got the message. I found the sharpest knife in the kitchen and spent half an hour shaving off the sides and base of the cake, in order to remove the paper without removing too much of the actual panforte. The result was a dessert that was smaller and less symmetrical than intended but at least edible—as long as you weren't wearing dentures.

With one bungle under my belt I was primed to expedite another. The main course was barbecued salmon and kingfish fillets, served with pomegranate and endive salad. I'd deliberately chosen something to which Dad could confidently contribute; he had a long history of manning the BBQ for my mother's dinner parties. I had never worked with pomegranates before, but the recipe was very straightforward, and why not try something new when potential in-laws were coming to dinner for the first time?

My father was curious. "Why pomegranates? Is it because Jewish tradition teaches that the pomegranate is a symbol of righteousness?" Daniel was Jewish. "Are you trying to give Daniel's family a subliminal message that you're righteous? They'll never fall for it. In Armenia pomegranates represent fertility, abundance and marriage. Is *that* your intention?"

"Look," I replied impatiently, "there's no hidden intention behind using pomegranates. They're in season, they're a bit exotic and the picture in the recipe book caught my eye."

I had no time for the mythology surrounding pomegranates. The recipe said to place a pomegranate on the bench and roll it around, pressing firmly with the palm of my hand. This would soften the fruit as the seeds released the juice. The final step was to slit the skin over a bowl and squeeze the juice out. I did exactly as instructed. I felt the fruit soften. It felt quite sensual … then suddenly—and this was not mentioned in the recipe—the fruit exploded! The skin burst, sending hundreds of bright pink pomegranate seeds into every corner of the kitchen. The seeds were accompanied by deep crimson juice, which splattered across the fridge, stove, walls, window sills, plates, cutlery, napkins and everything else I had put out for the meal. Not to mention our clothes. Luckily we were both wearing aprons. I looked at Dad in disbelief.

"Some Jewish scholars believe the pomegranate was the forbidden fruit in the Garden of Eden," he began to say.

"That's what you said about quinces!" I shouted.

"Different scholars believe different things. I believe the pomegranate should be forbidden fruit for *you*."

At least I had something to occupy my father for the next few hours. To his credit, he managed to remove most traces of the pomegranate eruption by the time the guests arrived. And I learnt to be gentle with the remaining pomegranates.

Packing: Take 1

Nature does not hurry, yet everything is accomplished.
Lao Tzu

The next time I went to Brisbane to present a series of workshops, I was too exhausted to organise three days' worth of meals, an encyclopaedia-length set of instructions and a team of chauffeurs and dad-sitters, so I decided to take Dad with me.

I was speaking on **Keeping Our Balance**, but it was the last thing I felt qualified to speak about. In the two months since my mother had died, I'd managed to lay claim to root canal therapy, cellulitis, headaches and recurrent sore throats—more health issues than I'd experienced during my entire life. Since I could not come at hypocrisy, I proposed to speak openly about how my life had been tipped *off* balance and what one could do to regain balance.

On the eve of our departure I handed my father a piece of paper with a list of what he was to pack. It would be an excellent, easy, confidence-boosting exercise for him. It would also tax him just a little, to make a few straightforward decisions about which of his 48 pairs of socks to take. Everything on the list was numbered in the order in which it should be packed; I didn't want bulky shoes crushing a lovingly ironed shirt. I looked forward to congratulating him on a job well done.

"We'll be leaving first thing in the morning, so you need to do this now," I told him. I left him and went to do my own packing. Fifteen minutes later, he was rummaging around one of his desk drawers. Nothing was in the suitcase.

"What are you doing?" I asked.

"I'm looking for spare batteries for my hearing aids," he replied.

"Are they playing up?" I queried.

"No, but how do I know they won't start playing up while we're away?"

"OK, but let's deal with contingencies after we've packed the basics. I'd like you to focus on the items on the list first."

I left him for another 15 minutes. When I returned he was sitting at the kitchen table sorting through papers. Two pairs of socks and two underpants lay crumpled in the suitcase.

"What are you doing *now*?" It took considerable effort to keep the volume of my voice to acceptable levels.

"There's a shop in Brisbane that sells inexpensive vitamins and memory supplements. I'm trying to find my customer number and the address of the store, so we can visit it."

"Can you do that *after* you've finished packing?"

"I've packed."

"You've *started* packing but you haven't *finished* packing. Do you think you could complete one task before you start another?"

"What do I need to pack?"

"It's on the list I gave you."

"Where's the list?"

"I don't know," I said through clenched teeth. "It was on the table the last time I saw it."

"How am I supposed to find it among all these other papers?"

"If you put the papers away, you'll find it." I was getting exasperated. He sighed and scrunched up his face, as though I'd just given him an unpalatable medicine. "The quicker you get this done," I bargained, "the sooner you'll be able to go back to your Sudoku." He reluctantly started putting away the papers.

I was terrified of checking on him another 15 minutes later. This time he was sitting in his favourite chair, with his Sudoku. The suitcase was a quarter packed and the list was nowhere in sight.

"OK, what's the story now?" My patience had reached its limit.

"I'm done."

"You're not done! Why are you being so uncooperative? What is so difficult about putting a few items in a suitcase?"

"I don't know what to pack! *Which* comfortable walking shoes do you want? *Which* trousers? *Which* short-sleeved blue shirt?"

"Whichever shoes *you* find most comfortable! Whichever blue shirt and trousers *you* want! It's not for me to make every single decision for you! How can you be so lazy and irresponsible? How dare you expect me to wait on you hand and foot!"

"If it's all too hard, go to Brisbane without me. I'll be more than happy here on my own," he sulked.

"It's not that it's too hard. I'd have packed your suitcase 10 times over by now. The point is for you to take some responsibility for your own life and to make decisions for yourself."

He said nothing. It slowly dawned on me that maybe I was asking too much of Dad. My mother had never allowed him to make his own decisions, even when he'd been capable. Following a list seemed a no-brainer to me, but it was probably more than his neural connections could handle. I said nothing more and finished packing his suitcase.

Tears

If you are pained by any external thing, it is not this thing that disturbs you, but your own judgment about it. It is in your power to wipe out this judgment now.
Marcus Aurelius

We were in a taxi on our way to the airport when Dad tapped me on the shoulder. At his insistence, I was sitting in the front seat, and he was diagonally behind me.

"I can't find my wallet," he announced.

"It's in your bag. I saw you put it in there just before we left home," I reassured him.

"It's not there now," he said evenly.

"Are you sure? Have you checked all the compartments?" I was certain he wouldn't have searched thoroughly enough.

"Yes."

"Do you mind if I have a look?"

"Go for it." He passed me his bag.

I unzipped every compartment and combed through all the contents. It wasn't there. What to do? If we turned back, we risked missing our flight. If we arrived without his ID, we risked him being refused a boarding pass. The longer I deliberated, the bleaker our prospects. I asked the driver to take us back home—so much for breakfast in the Qantas Club lounge.

Try as he might, the driver couldn't suppress his glee. "So you want me to go back to your home and then still take you to the airport?"

"Yes, and make it quick."

We were a few minutes from home when Dad tapped me on the shoulder again. "It's OK, I've found it."

"Where?" I turned around to glare at him.

"In my trouser pocket. I must have put it there for safekeeping and easy accessibility after I got in the taxi," he smiled.

"Driver, can you please head for the airport—again!"

At the airport, my father said I should tip the driver because he had accommodated our requests and "he seemed like a nice man".

"I'm a nice doctor and no one gives *me* a tip," I retorted, "and he didn't do us any favours. The meter was running the whole time. The fare is more than he expected—and more than *I* expected." I paid the exact fare and hurried to the check-in counter.

"Why not give him a tip?" Dad persisted while we queued. "Why not do something nice for someone when they least expect it? It would have made his day and taken nothing away from *your* day. If you die $5 richer or poorer, what difference will it make to your life? It's not about the money; it's about how he would've felt for the rest of the day. He would've passed those good feelings onto the next passenger and he would have gone home to his family and said, 'I had a good day today'. And you'd have contributed to his whole family being happy."

I was on the verge of tears but forced a smile for the woman at the check-in counter. She smiled back.

"You've been allocated exit row seats," she pronounced, "so I'll just have to change them."

I was taken aback. "Why? There's no need. I have a permanent request for an exit row seat in my frequent flyer profile."

"Yes, but Mr Popovic clearly can't remove a 20 kilogram door and throw it out of the aircraft," she said kindly.

"He won't need to," I assured her. "I'll be sitting in the window seat and *I'll* do it."

"I'm sorry. Everyone sitting in an exit row must be able to assist in the event of an emergency."

"But he'll be able to assist. I'll tell him exactly what to do," I guaranteed.

"I'm sorry. Everyone in an exit row seat needs to be fit and independently capable of whatever is required."

"Less than 15 per cent of Australians can be classified as fit," I countered. "You'll be struggling to fill those seats if that's your criterion."

"I'm sorry, I can't override policy and jeopardise the safety of other passengers on the plane." She handed me new seat allocations. "You'll have to go straight to the boarding gate. Your flight has already been called."

I burst into tears.

Dad stared at me. He wasn't used to displays of emotion from me, especially over something as trivial as an aircraft seat allocation. "Hey it's only a short flight. It doesn't matter where we sit," he tried to console me.

Of course it wasn't about the seats. It was about the packing, the wallet, the organising, the exhaustion and the unending list of things to do. It was about repeatedly thwarted plans. It was about the strain of motivating another human being, day in and day out, to take his next breath. It was about suppressed grief. And it was about the relentlessness of it all. My life was clearly out of balance.

Boundaries

No-one can drive us crazy unless we give them the keys.
Doug Horton

Everything was going to schedule and I was about to leave for my presentation. "I'll be back in a few hours," I called to Dad. I wrote the time of my return on a piece of paper and stuck it on the kitchen bench top.

"But I'm coming with you," he stated.

"No, not this time. It's an in-house talk and I'm only speaking for an hour. I haven't asked if I can bring you and it wouldn't be appropriate."

"Isn't that why you packed my suit? I'm ready to go." He emerged from his room looking quite dapper.

"No, the suit is for a dinner we're going to."

"But I want to hear you speak."

"You can come to all the Rotary talks I give."

Confession: I had started to schmooze all the Rotary Clubs in Sydney, systematically working through speaking engagements at every one of them. My motivation was shamefully self-serving: since I was always allowed to bring my father, it meant he would spend an evening in a stimulating environment, socialise with new people and get reinforcement of the brain-boosting messages I was giving him at home. Not to mention that it was a night off from cooking for me. If anyone reading this is a Rotarian, please forgive my utilitarian objectives—I was going through a hard time. I can honestly say I enjoyed all the meetings and would do it again, even without the father incentive.

"I want to go with you," Dad said.

"But it's so nice here. You've got the pool, the spa, the sauna, the balcony, the Serbian paper and Sudoku. You won't get through half of it by the time I'm back."

"I'd rather go with you." He looked crestfallen. "Then we can go down to the pool together." He never wanted to go anywhere and now on the one occasion he was requesting it, I was denying it. I felt the tears well up in my eyes again. What was going on with me lately?

"OK, let's go then," I relented. "I'll sort it out when we get there."

My client was very understanding and allowed Dad to sit in on the presentation. He was a completely unobtrusive presence in the audience—unlike my mother had been capable of being. When she'd attended a public workshop I'd given a year ago, she sat in the middle of the auditorium and used sign language to convey instructions on how to improve my delivery. *Get that strand of hair out of your eyes. Straighten your shoulders. Slow down. Don't wave your arms so much.* A mother has infinite ways of expressing her love.

When I was halfway through my presentation, I suddenly froze. I was about to launch into how recent circumstances had thrown my life out of balance. Yet there, looking at me expectantly, was my father. This was not something I wanted him to hear. I felt faint. I quickly asked my audience to turn to each other for a few minutes and recap what I'd covered thus far. Meanwhile I was going to be sick. My mind shuffled the rest of my material, but it simply wouldn't make sense without my personal example. I could feel the perspiration staining the underarms of my clothes, despite the heavy-duty deodorant. I took some long, slow, deep breaths. Then it came to me and I continued.

"Several years ago I found myself in a challenging relationship with a man and his two young children ..." I managed to transpose my current situation onto a past relationship and communicate the essence of the intended message. I seemed to get away with it.

While we were driving home, Dad said, "I never knew you'd had such a hard time with Nick and the kids. I'm pleased you've learnt to set boundaries and take better care of yourself now."

Jackfruit

Man who says "It cannot be done" should not interrupt
man who is doing it.
Chinese proverb

When my work in Brisbane was over, I treated my father to something he'd wanted to do for a long time. Seven years ago, on a holiday at Mission Beach, I went skydiving for the first time. I was so terrified that it took four men to pry my fingers off the edge of the plane, but once I was in freefall I loved it. I experienced such an adrenaline rush that after the jump I walked into the first real estate agent I found, asked to be shown some properties and promptly bought one. As you do.

Dad had always wanted to see my little beach house but my parents had never managed to get there. Mission Beach is a palm-lined piece of paradise in Far North Queensland, on the coast between Cairns and Townsville. We flew from Brisbane to Townsville, and then drove north in a hire car. We made the obligatory stop at Frosty Mango, a café and tropical fruit outlet, where I stocked up on brain-boosting breakfast ingredients.

The following morning, I was eager to taste the jackfruit we'd bought. Jackfruit is the largest tree fruit in the world, weighing up to 36 kilograms. It has a thick, brown, inedible covering which protects a sweet, yellow, fibrous bulb inside. My father had never heard of jackfruit, let alone eaten it. I felt excited about giving him a new sensory experience and proud that I didn't miss a single opportunity for brain boosting.

I'd eaten jackfruit in various parts of Southeast Asia, but I'd never had to cut one open. No-one had warned me that the sap, which oozed out as soon as I plunged the knife in, was the active ingredient of superglue. Before I realised what was happening, the chopping board had stuck to the knife, which had stuck to my hand, which had stuck to my shirt. I must have also got sap on my lips, because in my moment of greatest need, I found I was unable to open my mouth to call Dad for help.

I needn't have worried—the fact that I'd been silent for three minutes alerted my father that something was wrong. Just as it seemed that amputation was the only option, we stumbled upon a bottle of vinegar, which when mixed with dishwashing detergent and olive oil dissolved enough sap off my lips to allow me to speak. It took the next two days to remove all traces of sap from the bench top, fridge door, sink, taps and oven. I don't know how it managed to make its way to the toilet seat, but the patch of skin missing from my left buttock suggested that the sap had pervaded every aspect of our existence.

Despite my property requiring major repairs, a new coat of paint and new tenants, Dad loved it. He could only see the positives. He met the builder, he helped me select the colour scheme, and he chose the bougainvillea that would line the balcony. Sometimes I enjoyed having a constant companion.

Contribution

*The more sand that has escaped from the hourglass of our life,
the more clearly we should see through it.*
Niccolo Machiavelli

My father needed more than mateship; he needed meaning.

"I don't see the point of pure amusement," he grumbled. "For life to have any meaning, a person needs to be giving something of value to the world."

"But going to Men's Shed and Probus is contributing to the group and helping to create a supportive community," I urged. "Your presence is something of value."

Dad remained unconvinced, so my mission needed to expand to mateship and meaning, people and purpose, connection and contribution. Hello, Meals on Wheels!

"Meals on Wheels provides nutritionally-balanced meals to frail, aged people, who are unable to cook or shop for themselves and would otherwise be forced to live in a nursing home. You'll be doing a major community service," I implored my father, as we drove to the Meals on Wheels office.

"I'm too old for something like that." It was his usual response.

"You know, I'm really starting to lose patience with you. First you tell me you want to contribute to others, but when the opportunity presents itself you come up with some lame excuse to get out of it. Someone else will do the driving, and all you have to do is take the food from the car to the front door and check if there's anything else needed. For some people it's the only social contact they have all day—just a few minutes of your time. I find that very sad."

"If it's such an invaluable service, why aren't *you* volunteering?" he challenged.

"Because the work I do is already contributing to others. Not that I'm getting any time for work these days."

"Work is different; you get paid for that," he asserted. I was too angry to respond. "When will you get it through your head that old age imposes physical and mental limitations that render a person far less energetic and capable than they once were?" he maintained.

"When will you get it through *your* head," I retorted, "that old age doesn't have to be that way? The things you tell me about old age are just stories running around in your head. Have you heard of Frank Lloyd Wright?"

"Of course I have. He was America's greatest architect. He designed the Guggenheim Museum in New York."

"That's right. And do you know how old he was when he did that? He was 90! Nine zero when he designed one of the architectural icons of the twentieth century," I contended.

"There are always exceptions."

"There are a lot of exceptions—which means they aren't exceptions. They're an indication of what we're all capable of. Julia Britton in her late nineties is still a highly successful Australian playwright, with three plays produced last year. Eleanor Benz, a 90 year-old Chicago woman who dropped out of high school to help her family during the Great Depression, recently went back to school and attained her diploma, with 37 great-grandchildren to cheer her on. John Walker at age 86 completed his twenty-fifth Sydney to Hobart yacht race in 2008. Benjamin Franklin invented bifocal glasses at age 78.

Queenslander Betty Birsky published two award-winning books, *Homeland* and *At the Island*, at age 79 and 82 respectively, and she's now giving talks on her books and on writing. Edward de Bono, the originator of lateral thinking, has written seven books since turning 70. I heard him speak at a conference recently and he's as brilliant as ever. Ridley Scott, Britain's most successful film director in Hollywood, is in his seventies and was recently ranked number 35 in a list of the world's 100 most powerful people. I can keep going," I threatened.

"I know you can but as we've just arrived at Meals on Wheels, we'd better go in."

I would not be silenced. "Your mate, Dean, is 75 years old, plays tennis every day and is the biggest flirt I've ever come across."

Inside the building, I completed Dad's registration form. He immediately handed me another one. "This one's for you," he said. "If *you* don't do it, *I'm* not doing it."

I cast a wan smile at the receptionist.

"It would be lovely if you and your father did it together," she chirped. "How gorgeous: a father–daughter team!" I wanted to strangle her. Within a week we were ordained as the new father–daughter team. I was the driver and Dad was the runner. Tony was assigned to accompany us on our first run. He was 93 years old and had been a Meals on Wheels volunteer for more than 10 years.

"You've got a long career ahead of you!" I gloated at my father.

The following week we were on our own. In addition to the frozen meals, there was a bag of apples to distribute between the households. I'd slept in and missed breakfast, and half way through our run I was so hungry I would've eaten one of the meals had they not been frozen. That's when I remembered the apples. "We've been forgetting to hand out the apples!"

"Then we'll have to retrace our steps," Dad said.

Fabulous—it would be even longer before I got breakfast. But it was evident something had touched my father. "Why don't these people have family to look after them?" he asked pensively. "It's distressing to see the circumstances some people live in."

Over time a pattern emerged: my father was acutely sensitive to the plight of the lonely. "The more people there are in the world, the more loneliness there seems to be. It doesn't make sense," he observed. Dad believed that loneliness was the heaviest cross anyone could be made to bear. Whenever we visited people who lived alone, he felt the day had been worthwhile. I sent emails to friends and neighbours, asking if they knew companionless people who'd appreciate his company. We drove from one end of Sydney to the other, having coffee with widows and widowers. I gave us the codename "Mobile Mates".

Community

*I grieve the loss of old friends, only to find comfort
in the love of new friends.*
Glen Herrington-Hall

My mother's funeral showed me the meaning of community. She had worked at the same hospital for 38 years. Everyone who had ever been part of that community—trainee doctors, specialists, nurses, dieticians, physios, pharmacists, social workers, wardsmen, administrators, switchboard operators, cleaning staff and cooks—could remember when she first started in her crisp, starched coat and broken English. They watched her give 100 per cent to every position she'd held, culminating in her appointment as Director of Clinical Services. They'd all experienced her kindness, generosity and fervour for justice. Most importantly, they knew she cared passionately about every one of them, patients and staff alike.

Because she belonged to the same community for so many years, her contributions were recognised and respected. She'd never have become an anonymous "old lady" in retirement because she belonged to people who shared almost four decades of memories.

In today's society we frequently move from one address, community and workplace to another. Personally, I find this interesting, exciting and fulfilling, but one of the costs of an itinerant lifestyle is erosion of reverence for the elderly. The old people we encounter aren't people we knew from our childhood or people we watched mould our community. They become the person who takes the longest time to cross the road and therefore holds us up when we're running late.

This disconnection, lack of recognition and feeling of social isolation was why my maternal grandfather returned to Serbia within a few years of arriving in Australia. He had been a vet in Vršac and was known to everyone in town. Even after he was no longer formally working, people would bring their horses to him for attention. During the day he'd sit out on his front porch and every passer-by would stop to talk, often staying for hours, playing cards and sharing meals.

So when he came to Australia, my grandfather put two cane chairs on our front porch, made himself comfortable in one of them and waited to greet the passers-by. There were none. And the few who walked past hardly turned their heads; they certainly showed no interest in conversation or cards. My grandfather was bitterly disenchanted with the Promised Land and insisted that my parents buy him a ticket back home. But his wife (my grandmother) had become a popular figure in my school community and opted to stay. I think he believed she would change her mind and join him but she didn't. They only saw each other one more time during the remaining 30 years of their lives.

Appreciation

A faithful friend is the medicine of life.
Unknown, though often attributed to the Bible

Whether it was the goji berries in the panforte or just general wear and tear, Dad's dentures had become uncomfortably loose and needed adjusting, so we made an appointment to see his denture maker.

It was love at first sight. Dennis the denturist was everything I wanted—for my father. He was a chatty, cheerful, cheeky 81 year-old, who loved his work and boasted that he'd sent six Valentine's Day cards this year (one more than last year). He was motivated and goal-oriented and had no intention of retiring in the foreseeable future. "Why on earth would I?" he asked rhetorically. "I'm doing a lot of good for a lot of people."

I responded by quoting research confirming that people who lived sociable, purposeful lives improved their longevity and had a much lower risk of depression and dementia.

"If you're doing something that benefits others," Dennis reasoned, "you can't get depressed and you can't afford to get dementia. That's commonsense. You don't need research to tell you that. 'Thank you' is the best medicine on the planet—I'll bet they didn't teach you *that* in medical school."

I wanted Dennis to become my father's best mate. Dennis would have a very positive influence on Dad. Dennis would be my answer to Marko.

I batted my eyelids and smiled sweetly as I sat supportively by my father's side. I fantasised about Dennis and Dad going to the movies together; Dennis and Dad playing lawn bowls together;

Dennis and Dad going out to lunch together; and Dennis and Dad chatting up women together. I sighed in contentment.

When we returned the next day to pick up the repaired dentures, I took Dennis a bottle of wine.

"What's this for?" He looked pleasantly surprised.

"You said it was the best medicine on the planet … ," I replied bashfully.

When we were outside, my father shook his head. "Anyone would think you had a crush on that man."

"Don't be ridiculous. I wanted to show our appreciation. You're the one who keeps telling me to give people tips."

He eyed me suspiciously. "Well, just remember that he's old enough to be your father. Actually, he's older!"

I started plotting how we might get Dennis to our place for a meal.

Part IV
Changing His Mind

*The greatest risk a man can take is not to aim too high and miss,
but to aim too low and hit.*

Michelangelo

Panacea

Old age isn't so bad when you consider the alternative.
Maurice Chevalier

"I have a present for you," I smiled, handing Dad a small, square box wrapped in blue paper with a gold ribbon.

"Oh? What is it?" he asked indifferently.

"It's the closest thing there is to a panacea." My father raised his eyebrows, but I continued. "You know I don't believe in wonder drugs or quick fixes, but this is the most potent medicine on the planet for improving brain function and preventing disease."

He looked even more incredulous. "Aren't I taking enough medications already? What does my GP say about this?"

"Both your GP and your psychiatrist think it's essential," I confirmed.

"Is it new?" he probed.

"It's been around for a long time but scientists have only recently discovered the extent of its benefits."

"How long do I have to take it for?"

"Every day for the rest of your life, just like your heart and memory tablets."

"Then it isn't a gift," he sighed and began untying the ribbon.

"Absolutely it's a gift. I couldn't give you a greater gift—I'm giving you the gift of life, of vitality, energy and wellbeing! But before you open it, sit down and I'll tell you exactly what it will do for you."

"Go ahead, knock yourself out," he replied wearily.

"Every benefit has been backed by extensive research of the highest calibre: randomised, controlled trials (RCT), as well as far-reaching epidemiological studies," I declared.

"The side effects must be pretty bad if you're going to such huge lengths to convince me to take this," he contested.

"No, there are no side effects at all. Unless of course you overdose but I guarantee that won't happen. OK, here goes:

- It induces the formation of new brain cells.
- It improves memory and concentration.
- It cuts our lifetime risk of dementia in half.
- It reduces the risk of Alzheimer's Disease by over 60 per cent.
- It lowers the risk of cancer, including colon and breast cancer, which are the two most prevalent cancers in men and women respectively.
- It lowers the risk of cardiovascular disease, including heart attack and stroke.
- It strengthens the immune system.
- It prevents Type 2 diabetes and helps mitigate the effects of Type 1 diabetes.
- It reduces the risk of bone loss (osteoporosis) by increasing bone mineral density.
- It reduces the number of falls and fall-related fractures in the elderly by 35 per cent.
- It has an anti-depressant effect equivalent to that of Prozac and reduces the risk of developing depression in the first place by up to 50 per cent.
- It dissipates stress and counteracts the negative effects of stress on the body.
- It boosts our energy levels.

- It improves strength and stamina.
- It promotes better sleep and is helpful for insomnia.
- It aids slimming if you need to lose weight and helps maintain weight loss once you've lost weight.
- It lifts self-esteem and enhances sexual libido."

"Oh great—just what I need!"

"I included that last one for completeness," I grinned. "The bottom line is that if everyone took this medicine, the Australian health care system could conservatively save $1.5 billion a year. That's almost one-fifth of our total health care costs. Go ahead. Open it."

Dad took meticulous care removing the wrapping and then turned the box over in his hands, trying to make sense of the picture on it. He shook his head and lifted the lid. "I still don't know what it is."

"It's a pedometer, an instrument that records the number of steps you take."

He still looked bewildered.

"The single most important thing you can do to boost your brain and extend your life is to move your body, to **run the motor**," I explained. "If we don't engage in physical activity, both our bodies and brains waste away. Your target is to walk 10 000 steps every day."

"You must be joking," my father replied.

"I have never been more serious. If this was a century ago we wouldn't be having this conversation because 100 years ago Australians were walking 16 kilometres every day, just in the course of their normal activities. *You'd* be lucky to walk one kilometre a day. Humans were designed to walk, and our brains need us to move in order to develop properly and to remain in good working condition. As little as 20 minutes of exercise every second day cuts our lifetime risk of dementia in half and reduces our risk of Alzheimer's Disease by over 60 per cent! How phenomenal is that!? Bump it up to 20 minutes *every* day and we also cut our risk of stroke by 57 per cent. None of the medications you're taking come close to giving you the same benefits.

"There are piles and piles of research papers showing that a sedentary lifestyle is the greatest predictor of poor health and poor cognitive functioning as we age. One reason is that lack of exercise compromises blood flow to the heart and brain. Conversely, when we move, more oxygen and nutrients are delivered to the brain and more waste products are removed. Exercise also helps to lower blood pressure, lower inflammation and prevent obesity, all of which are independent risk factors for dementia. Whatever's good for the heart is also good for the brain. Specifically in relation to memory, exercise increases blood flow to a region of the hippocampus called the dentate gyrus. The more you exercise, the bigger your dentate gyrus and the better your memory.

"A Western Australian Centre for Health and Ageing study published in the *Journal of the American Medical Association* confirmed that a walk a day keeps memory loss away," I continued my lecture. "Conducted over 18 months, 170 participants aged over 50 who felt they had memory problems were divided into two groups. One group walked for 50 minutes three times a week or participated in another form of moderate exercise. The other group continued with their usual activities. The result was that the exercise group—even if they only walked 20 minutes a day—performed better at cognitive tasks, such as remembering lists of words.

"And the story gets better and better. As well as improving blood flow, exercise stimulates the production of a substance called brain-derived neurotrophic factor (BDNF), which is like a fertiliser for neurons. BDNF actually promotes the formation of new brain cells and connections between brain cells. And the more you exercise, the more BDNF you produce!"

As I paused for breath I could see an objection forming on Dad's lips. I got in first. "And you're never too old to experience the benefits of exercise! Your brain will respond to the increased blood flow and the presence of BDNF at any age: nine or 99 and any age in between. A study published in 2006 reported that those over age 60 who engaged in brisk walking for three hours a week over a six-month period increased both grey matter[1] and white matter[2] and enlarged their overall brain volume.

"Another way that exercise exerts brain-protective and anti-ageing effects is because it's a mild form of stress."

"You're certainly right about that!" Dad agreed.

"And that's a good thing." I motored straight on. "The stress of exercise causes our bodies to produce free radicals[3] that induce genes in muscles and neurons to make proteins that protect our cells from stress. It's a bit like getting a vaccination against the harmful effects of stress. Not to mention the fact that you'll simply feel better and have more energy throughout the day."

"How will I have more energy when you're going to make me *exert* energy?" my father protested.

---

1   Grey matter consists of nerve cell bodies, supporting cells and capillaries.
2   White matter contains myelinated nerve fibres called axons. Myelin acts as insulation and is composed largely of fatty tissue, which turns white when preserved in formaldehyde.
3   Free radicals are highly chemically reactive atoms or molecules believed to contribute to developing cancer and degenerative diseases.

"That's the greatest paradox of exercise: you have to exert some energy to get going, but you get it back tenfold for the rest of the day. And once you get fit, you'll start to enjoy it and look forward to it."

Dad was dubious.

"We'll start slowly," I reassured him, "and it has to be fun. If it isn't, your adrenal glands will produce cortisol, which is highly toxic to the brain so the whole thing will be counter-productive. That's why I have a second present for you."

"I'm not sure I like your presents."

I handed him a membership card to the local gym.

"No way!" he complained. "A gym is no place for a 78 year-old! Besides, I get enough physical exercise by hanging out the washing and doing all the other jobs you give me."

"Don't make me laugh," I countered. "The closest you've come to exercising around me is pushing your luck!"

Table Tennis

How old would you be if you didn't know how old you were?
Satchel Paige

"Let me read you something," I waved the newspaper at my father. "Dorothy De Low has been awarded a Medal of the Order of Australia for services to table tennis. Guess how old she is."

"How old?"

"She's celebrating her 100th birthday this year!"

"That's nice for her."

"That's an example of staying mentally and physically fit till the day you die!"

"OK, so the woman's been playing table tennis all her life and it's a familiar world to her," Dad claimed. "My situation is different. You're asking me to start a range of activities that are a whole new ballgame for me, if you'll excuse the pun."

"Well, just listen to this!" I exclaimed triumphantly. "Dorothy only started playing table tennis in her *seventies*! And she represented Australia at the World Veterans Table Tennis Championships when she was 78 years old—exactly your age. In 1992, when she was 81, she was the World Veteran Champion in the over 80s division. She says that not only does she enjoy playing the game, but it keeps her reflexes sharp and it's a great social outlet. And this is a woman who lives by herself only a few suburbs from here. She's managed to find meaning and joy in her life, despite her personal losses. I admire her immensely."

Whether Dad was aware of it or not, the constant barrage of healthy, successful agers was slowly opening his mind to new possibilities for himself.

Ally

A man without a goal is like a boat without a rudder.
Thomas Carlyle

Dad's pedometer became my best friend and ally. Clipping it to his belt every morning was motivation for him to achieve something. It operated as a subliminal commitment to his wellbeing and demonstrated that it was within his capacity to make a difference. Although he regularly objected to the "ordeal", I could see that he felt a sense of accomplishment at reaching his target number of steps for the day.

The pedometer was sending my father a message that he was doing something positive for himself and that he was taking responsibility for his mental and physical health. We started with 1 000 steps a day—just over one kilometre—and week by week, gradually increased the distance. The pedometer was also an objective indicator of his progress. I used it as a reference point to remind him that he was not too old to reach new milestones.

On alternate days we went to the gym together. We varied our workouts, so that in the course of a week my father's fitness regime included weight training, pilates, rowing and yoga.

"Why do I have to go to the gym as well as walk? Isn't the walking enough?"

"Walking is excellent, but you get an added brain-boosting effect if your exercise challenges your balance and coordination and involves both sides of your body and all four limbs. Movements that intersect the midline, where one limb crosses to the opposite side, are particularly good for your brain. The more complex and challenging the movements, the better. Also the benefits increase when you exercise in company."

"Even annoying company?" he teased.

"Yes, Dad, even annoying company. Ideally, I'd have you taking dance classes. In a 21-year study of senior citizens, people who regularly danced were 76 per cent less likely to develop dementia. Dancing ticks so many boxes when it comes to boosting the brain: it involves balance, coordination, memory, new skill acquisition and social stimulation. We'll get to it in time …"

Triumph

The only person you're destined to become
is the person you decide to be.
Ralph Waldo Emerson

One day a young woman approached me at the gym. "Excuse me, are you a personal trainer?"

"No, I'm not," I replied.

"Oh, it's just that I see you working with that elderly gentleman and I wondered if you'd take on my mother as a client."

"That's my father."

"How lovely!" She was genuinely delighted. "It's so inspiring watching him. I've told my mum about this 70-something year-old man who works out at the gym, and she's slowly coming around to the idea of doing something herself. I've told her age is no excuse for not exercising. The older we get, the more important it is to keep moving."

"Absolutely," I concurred. "A lot of older people find a gym intimidating because they're afraid they won't know what to do or how to use the equipment. But if you offer to show her and get her started, it'll make her feel less self-conscious and you can get her a personal trainer when she's feeling more confident."

"Thank you!" she smiled brightly and returned to her Stair-Master.

I bounded over to Dad. "How about that?" I offhandedly remarked.

"How about what?"

"You're an inspiration to that young woman and her mother."

"Don't be ridiculous."

"She just told me so. She's going to bring her mother to the gym, which will increase the quality and longevity of her mother's life—all thanks to you. Can't you see that simply doing your thing—being *you*—is reason for you to live? You're making a positive difference to others whether you like it or not!"

Night Cap

*The person who knows how to laugh at himself
will never cease to be amused.*
Shirley MacLaine

The faint tap on the front door came at 11 pm. Before I let my visitor in, I tiptoed down the darkened hallway and checked the status of Dad's bedroom lamp. It was off. My father was breathing slowly and rhythmically, flirting with the idea of snoring. I carefully closed all the doors that separated his bedroom from mine. I glided back down the hallway and let my patient guest inside.

We were finally alone in my bedroom. Just to be safe, I kept the lights off. It had been such a long time, we felt like strangers to each other. We slid under the Bugs Bunny doona. Our clothes took languid turns flying out onto the floor as we began re-acquainting ourselves with each other's contours. Our eyes slowly adjusted to the darkness.

Suddenly my bedroom was ablaze with light. Daniel dived under the covers with Road Runner swiftness. I sat up, blinking at my father and holding my breath.

"Something woke me up," he stated matter-of-factly.

"You must've had a disturbing dream, Dad," I confidently proposed.

"Maybe … I can't remember. Just thought I'd check that you were OK."

"I'm perfectly fine, thanks, Dad. You can go back to sleep."

"OK. Goodnight then." He closed the door and indolently shuffled back to his room.

Dan cautiously emerged for air. "I feel like a 16 year-old."

"What?" I responded with mock dismay. "You were sneaking into the homes of girlfriends at the age of 16?"

Juggling

The moment one gives close attention to anything, even a blade of grass, it becomes a mysterious, awesome, indescribably magnificent world in itself.
Henry Miller

The benefits of physical exercise aren't just long-term. Movement brings immediate improvement in alertness, attention and cognition.

German researchers found that people learnt new words 20 per cent faster after exercise than they did before exercise, and the rate of learning correlated directly with increased levels of BDNF. In another experiment, 35 minutes on a treadmill at brisk walking pace improved processing speed and creative thinking for over an hour afterwards. Japanese scientists found that exercising only two to three times a week for 12 weeks improved what's known as executive brain function: decision making, problem solving, goal setting and extrapolation.

In 2004, researchers at Leeds Metropolitan University in England found that workers who used the company gym at lunchtime for 30–60 minutes, doing an aerobic class, weights or yoga, were more productive and felt better able to handle their workloads. Other studies show that employees who exercise regularly have fewer sick days and are better able to focus on their work.

Even just 12 minutes of exercise is enough to get our endorphins[4] flowing and to pick up our mood. On my father's reluctant days, I only asked 12 minutes of him. More often than not,

---

4   Endorphins (a fusion of *endogenous* and *morphine*) are the body's own pain-killers and pleasure chemicals. The brain produces them during excitement, injury, spicy food consumption and orgasm, as well as exercise.

after 12 minutes he was feeling agreeable enough to do another 12 minutes, so we managed to get his daily dose in after all.

Each time we came home from a walk or workout, I'd teach my father to juggle! One ball, then two balls and eventually three. One study showed that five weeks of juggling lessons increased the size of certain parts of the brain by 5 per cent. However, the main purpose of teaching Dad to juggle was to help him focus. **Focus is the magic bullet when it comes to preserving brain function and boosting brain performance.** And focus was my father's biggest struggle. He could not focus long enough to order Thai takeaway. His attention kept wandering from the menu, and even when I sat with him and talked him through it, by the time I explained what was in one dish, he'd forgotten what was in the previous one, so we had to start from the beginning.

Our ability to focus and learn new information is at its best in the first hour after aerobic exercise, so it was an ideal time to challenge him. Whether or not he ever learnt to juggle three balls didn't matter. What I was really training him to do was to pay attention, to get out of his comfort zone and to break his habit of living on autopilot. Boredom, sameness and stereotypical behaviours are poison for our brains.

To rescue our brains from decline, we need to continue challenging ourselves, to tackle new terrain and to conquer new frontiers. Crossword puzzles and Sudoku are good little brain boosters but they aren't enough. We need to get adventurous, get exploring and get out of our routines. We need to **sail to new shores.** We do our brains a big favour every time we do things differently and actively learn new things—and **active learning** means more than passively watching a TV documentary. There is nothing wrong with watching documentaries but they simply don't stimulate our brains in the same way as learning a foreign language, a musical instrument, an art, a craft, a skill or a sport.

Learning something new in old age, such as playing the piano, enhances our overall mental performance because the learning process itself improves communication between brain cells. High mental activity after retirement is associated with a 40–50 per cent reduction in the risk of dementia. We need to practise intense concentration and absorption, like we did automatically when we were children. Our brains thrive on it. While we're toddlers, going to school, studying at university, learning a trade or coming to grips with a new job, the brain is engaged in continuous skill acquisition and exacting learning. But once we settle into a job and get comfortable, our learning drops off dramatically, even if we regularly upgrade our skills. **Once we've learnt the ropes, we need to learn something else.** Our brains need to be dealing with unfamiliar undertakings on an ongoing basis, not just in the first half of our lives. Lifelong, exigent learning is the recipe for a sharp mind until the end of our days.

The power of intense, active learning lies in the fact that it requires us to pay close attention; we have to **focus on the present moment**. Intense focus has the same effect on our brains that lifting weights has on our muscles: it changes the brain's structure, strengthens connections between brain cells and increases the brain's capacity for long-lasting learning. Deliberately focusing our attention on a task—that means *not* multi-tasking and not doing things mindlessly—increases our processing speed, our effectiveness and our intelligence.

Although we are capable of multi-tasking we are not capable of multi-focusing: neither the male nor the female brain can focus on more than one thing at a time. If we're doing three things at once, the brain is rapidly switching focus from one activity to the next. This greatly reduces our efficiency and increases the likelihood of oversights and mistakes.

When we're not focused, it's as though we're working in a poorly lit room. With practice we get reasonably skilled at fumbling around in the dark, but we never reach our potential. On the other hand, when we pay full attention to what we're doing, it's like suddenly switching on the lights and seeing clearly — the task becomes much easier and our performance inevitably improves. If we learn something in an environment where other things are competing for our attention, we don't remember for very long. If we're fully focused on something, we remember for much longer because we create lasting changes in the brain.

The explanation for focus being such a powerful brain booster lies in a collection of acetylcholine-rich neurons in the basal forebrain called the nucleus basalis of Meynert, which I'll call NBOM for short. When the NBOM is turned on, as it is from birth to early childhood, it allows us to focus our attention and to remember what we're experiencing. The result of a switched-on NBOM is effortless learning and performing at our peak, which is why children learn things more quickly than adults.

A switched-on NBOM secretes acetylcholine, a neurotransmitter that helps us concentrate and form distinct memories. Conversely, people with a cognitive impairment produce less acetylcholine. This was the reason Dad had such difficulty focusing: he was *biologically incapable* of paying attention because his brain wasn't producing enough acetylcholine. However, if I could get him to focus on something, it would turn on his acetylcholine production. It was a chicken and egg scenario — acetylcholine enables us to focus and focusing enables us to produce acetylcholine. It seemed like a cruel dilemma: the solution to Dad's problem was for him to do the very thing his problem stopped him from being able to do. My only hope was to find things that naturally grabbed his attention without him having to make a conscious effort.

The NBOM is turned on during what is known as the "critical period" in brain development. During this time, simply being exposed to new stimuli can change the structure of our brains, which is why babies learn to speak just by hearing adults speak. An activated NBOM turns the brain into a sponge, absorbing information from everywhere. We learn what is safe, what causes pain, what leads to reward and what works in getting our needs met. We learn basic survival skills. And we learn all this with incredible ease because the NBOM is automatically and permanently turned on—we can't help but take everything in.

It is the presence of brain-derived neurotrophic factor (BDNF) during the critical period that keeps the NBOM turned on. As we grow, the NBOM is switched on less and less because we no longer need to absorb everything from our environment. We've mastered some essential skills, so we can afford to be more selective about what to pay attention to. When we've learnt to negotiate effectively with the world around us, it's BDNF again that turns *off* the NBOM. From that time on, probably around the age of eight years old, the NBOM is only turned on when:

- Something of great consequence or significance occurs.
- We face something entirely new or unexpected.
- We're totally fascinated or excited by something and we love doing it, so our attention is naturally absorbed by the task.
- We make a conscious effort to pay close attention and to be totally focused.

Exposing ourselves to the above situations is the key to keeping our brains in top shape for the duration of our lives.

This also highlights why the NBOM is turned on more often in children than in adults: children find more things intriguing, surprising and deserving of their full attention than do adults. However, as adults, we can turn on the NBOM by giving ourselves new challenges and by making a conscious effort to be fully focused on whatever we're doing.

The result of a turned-on NBOM is rapid learning and feeling "in flow". Athletes refer to this high performance state as "being in the zone", but it's a state available to all of us if we learn to pay attention. A critical point is that it's difficult for us to continue paying attention to something if there's no intrinsic reward or pleasure in doing so. Therefore, fun and positive feedback are important in helping to sustain our attention. The key message is to continue seeking out things that not only challenge us, but which we enjoy doing and find ourselves getting completely immersed in. The good news is that the more we practise focusing, the easier it becomes and the more we improve and maintain our overall mental function and memory.

Eggs

Death is a challenge. It tells us not to waste time ... It tells us to tell each other right now that we love each other.
Leo F. Buscaglia

Three months after my mother died, I had to give a series of presentations in Brisbane and decided that Dad was ready for the challenge of spending two days on his own. Of course I left a paper trail through the fridge to show what food was to be eaten at which meal on which day, and how it needed to be heated or assembled.

Just as I was about to give my first presentation, I remembered that I hadn't switched off my mobile phone. I pulled it out of my bag at the very moment a call came through from my father. Not *now*. I hesitated—if I didn't answer, I'd be wondering the entire time I was speaking why Dad had rung me. I took the call.

"You've put two eggs in a little container in the fridge and all you've written on the container is 'Boil these two eggs for lunch on Tuesday and add to the ingredients in container #2.' How do I boil the eggs? I mean, I know you put them in a saucepan on the stove, but for how long? Do I start timing from the time I switch the stove on or from the time the water starts boiling? Do you boil the water first and then drop the eggs in or do you place the eggs in cold water? Do you cover the saucepan with a lid or do you leave the lid off?"

I answered each question in turn before running onto the stage. When I turned my phone back on later, there were no missed calls, so I presumed all had gone well. In the evening I rang to check how Dad's day had been and how he'd managed with the eggs.

"Oh, I couldn't remember what you said after I hung up, so I did something even better: I ate the cake you'd left me to snack on."

"How was that better?"

"Well, when you made the cake I saw you put eggs in it, plus a whole lot of other ingredients. So the cake was better nutrition because I was eating eggs as well as flour and nuts and fruit and whatever else was in it. You're always saying I need to get as many different foods into my diet as I can."

"Yes, you're right, that's something I'm always saying. I'm impressed with your initiative."

The evening of my return home, I talked him through boiling four eggs. I noted what time he'd put them on, but told him that he was responsible for switching off the stove and removing the saucepan when they were done. I went to check my email in the next room.

"I'm just taking the eggs off now," he called out at exactly the right time. Who says you can't teach an old dog new tricks?

A few minutes later I went to the kitchen to inspect the eggs. Dad had resumed his Sudoku. Something was amiss. I removed my glasses, gave them a wipe and took another look. It wasn't possible.

"Dad, correct me if I'm wrong, but are these eggs *blue*?"

"Yes, they are," he smiled. "I think they look very pretty. I remembered something your grandmother used to do, which you've obviously forgotten. Whenever she boiled eggs she'd place a piece of cloth on the bottom of the saucepan and sit the eggs on top to stop them from cracking. If the eggs are in contact with the metal base or sides of the saucepan, the heat is likely to make them crack. This way we have perfect, uncracked eggs."

"I see. And so they're blue because the piece of cloth you used was blue and the dye has dyed the eggs."

"Yes. Shame we didn't do it at Easter. There are plenty of cloths of all different colours in the laundry."

"Yes, but cloth dye is not the same as food colouring. It's just possible we might poison ourselves if we eat these eggs."

"Nonsense. The eggs aren't cracked, so none of the dye would have seeped through the shell."

I was so tired that I didn't care if we *did* poison ourselves. But obviously I survived to tell the story.

Ambidexterity

Small things can make a big difference. Just try going to sleep with a mosquito in the room.
African proverb

Given the overly busy, frantic, deadline-ridden and exhausting lives that many people lead, who has time to learn a foreign language for no other reason than to boost the brain? Clearly, when we're at the height of our productivity and income-earning capacity, our priorities are maximum gain in minimum time. We need brain-boosting practices that can easily be incorporated into our "mandatory" daily activities. (I say "mandatory" because everything we do is ultimately a choice, even if we don't recognise that we've made a choice. Often our choice is based on an unconscious assessment that the cost of *not* doing something outweighs the cost or benefits of doing the thing.) Simply changing our routine and doing habitual things differently can help to keep our thinking sharp and our creativity flowing. Here are some suggestions:

- Take a shower with your eyes closed.
- Practise ambidexterity. Brush your teeth or use your computer mouse with the opposite hand to usual. Teach yourself to write with your non-dominant hand.
- Go to work via a new route, or walk the children to school a different way. Don't always take the same roads.
- Use a street directory instead of the GPS (Shock! Horror!).
- Engage in conversations with people you don't know.
- Find a new word in the dictionary at the start of each week and weave it into your conversations until it becomes a permanent part of your vocabulary.
- Listen to music that's different to what you're in the habit of listening to. (If your neighbours inflict on you their noise pollution, you can thank them for boosting your brain.)

Altering routines and habits requires us to snap out of being on autopilot and to start paying attention to what we're doing. It means we practise turning on the NBOM and begin to live more in the moment. Dad and I enjoyed learning to write with our non-dominant hands, which for both of us was our left. It made perfect sense to him that ambidexterity could improve his cognition, and he approached the exercise with surprising enthusiasm. This made it a double win: focus *and* fun.

Stillness

The quieter you become, the more you can hear.
Ram Dass

I believe the NBOM is where science and spirituality meet.

Many spiritual practices turn on the NBOM because they ask us to focus our attention: on our breathing, on what we're feeling in our bodies, on a candle flame, on a single visual point or on the present moment. Meditation and mindfulness are the two most obvious examples.

In the Bible, Jesus says, "I tell you the truth, unless you change and become like little children, you will never enter the kingdom of heaven. Therefore, whoever humbles himself like this child is the greatest in the kingdom of heaven." Becoming "like little children" means approaching the world with wonder, curiosity, freshness and delight. It means being inquisitive and asking hundreds of questions every day. It means having an insatiable appetite for learning. It means being totally absorbed in play and living in the present moment. It means turning on the NBOM.

Learning about the NBOM, as well as research supporting the physical, psychological and emotional benefits of meditation, was what finally convinced me to spend 10 to 20 minutes a day "doing nothing". It turns out that this particular form of doing nothing was doing a great deal: sharpening my mind, strengthening my immune system, increasing my energy levels, and enabling me to deal with my father much more calmly and effectively. The most powerful time to meditate is first thing on waking and immediately before sleep. It sets an uplifting tone for the day and settles the mind in preparation for slumber.

Stilling the mind is as important as stimulating the mind. If we don't use it, we lose it, but **if we never stop, we drop.** Stopping means not only relaxing our bodies but also **pressing the pause button** on our thinking. Formal meditation is one way to achieve this.

A *Time* magazine article described meditation as "the smart person's bubble bath", and smart people are definitely taking it up. Meditation is offered in schools, prisons, hospitals, law firms, and government and corporate offices. Outside Australia, there are dedicated "meditation rooms" in airports, alongside the duty free shops and Internet kiosks.

What exactly is meditation and how do we go about it? Meditation is a group of mental practices that people have engaged in for millennia to achieve spiritual, psychological and physical goals. What the practices have in common, or at least aim towards, is the experience of mental silence. Simply put, meditation is being in a state of mental quietness, where we aren't caught up in the constant noise of thinking. We're completely alert, aware and focused on the present moment, but we aren't actually thinking about anything.

I struggled to comprehend this notion, as I'd always lived by Descartes' pronouncement, "I think, therefore I am". How is it possible not to think?

Take a break from reading and try the following exercise. You may like to record yourself reading the instructions or do it in small chunks, as it's a lot to remember in one go.

Start by looking at the palm of your hand. Don't comment, criticise, judge or mentally describe what you see. Don't start to have a conversation with yourself—"Is that my lifeline? Wow, I'm going to live for ages!" Drop all that. Simply look without thinking. If a thought crosses your mind, just let it pass and bring your attention back to your hand. Either focus on one point or scan your entire palm, whichever you prefer.

After a minute, close your eyes and listen. Become aware of the different sounds around you, inside the room or outside in the street. You might hear the whir of an air-conditioner, the traffic on the road, or the song of a bird. Or just become aware of the silence.

Keeping your eyes closed, become aware of everything you're touching: the clothes on your skin, the shoes on your feet, the glasses on your nose and the chair against your back.

Now become aware of any bodily sensations, independent of what you're touching. Starting with your feet and working your way up, slowly scan your body for any tingling, discomfort, warmth or pain, all the way to the crown of your head. Go at your own pace and, once again, don't mentally describe the experience to yourself—just experience it.

Finally, become aware of your breathing. Feel the breath entering your nose or mouth, filling your lungs, expanding your chest and then leaving. Notice the pause between inhaling and exhaling. Feel your body relax as you exhale. Take several deep, slow, deliberate breaths and follow the air all the way in and all the way out. Then open your eyes.

Did you find that you were able to switch off your thinking because you were purely looking, listening or feeling? If not for the entire time, then at least for some of the time? These techniques are all ways of pressing the pause button on our thinking. They don't require any special environment or training, and even a minute can have a rejuvenating effect on the brain and body. How so?

Take a jar and fill a quarter of it with sand and three quarters with water. Replace the lid and let it stand. When the jar is still, the sand settles to the bottom and the water is clear. If you pick up the jar and shake it, the sand swirls around and the water becomes murky. The water represents the mind and the grains of sand are our thoughts. If we have thoughts flying around in our heads every waking hour, where's the space for creativity? Where's the silence that allows us to hear our intuition? If we press the pause button on our thinking, even just for a minute, we not only create space for clarity, we also allow our subconscious resources to come to the fore.

Meditative Moments, as I call the exercises above, allow us to settle the sand. The phrase "come to your senses" has a powerful double meaning.

When we keep our brains constantly busy, especially with input from computers, we forfeit mental downtime that allows us to learn better, retain new information and generate fresh ideas. When rats learn to navigate a new maze, their brains show a specific, new pattern of electrical stimulation. From then on, whenever they go through the maze, their neurons fire in the same way to create the same pattern. When the rats take a nap after their learning, their brains continue to replay the new pattern of firing while they sleep. However, if their rest is interrupted, or if they continue to be stimulated with different activities, they have trouble remembering how to get through the maze the following day. The same thing occurs in humans.

We need time out from mental stimulation to enable our brains to review experiences, consolidate them and turn them into concrete memories. A University of Michigan study found that people learned significantly better after a walk in nature than a walk in a crowded urban environment, implying that continual processing of rousing information is mentally draining. Sending SMSs while standing in a supermarket queue (a favourite, former pastime of mine) might feel like we're making good use of wasted time, but we're robbing ourselves of valuable cerebral respite. We'd actually give our brains a boost if we stood quietly in the queue, focusing on our breathing, or just tuning in to what's going on in our bodies.

This was something my father had been telling me for decades. It was an area of brain boosting where he was years ahead of me.

Meditation

When you lose touch with inner stillness,
you lose touch with yourself.
Eckhart Tolle

After I'd begun to integrate Meditative Moments into my day and became less reactive, better able to concentrate and more productive as a result, I decided to tackle formal meditation. Sitting still and not entertaining a barrage of thoughts did not come naturally to me, so I figured I'd take myself to a local meditation class—but not before I'd turned meditation into a methodical, intellectual pursuit. I failed to see the irony of this at the time.

With so many different meditation schools, surely I needed to investigate all of them before making a decision? I wouldn't want to be taught the wrong pose or mantra, or given the wrong prayer beads, if a pose, mantra or prayer beads were indeed necessary.

The primary purpose of meditation over most of its history has been to achieve spiritual goals. In most Buddhist traditions, the aim of meditation is to attain nirvana (enlightenment) or freedom from suffering. Other religions see prayer and meditation as two-way communication with God: when a person prays, *they* talk and God listens; when a person meditates, *God* talks and the person listens. Warriors of the ancient world used meditation to prepare for battle. In today's corporate world, meditation is being used as a stress management tool, while many performers and athletes meditate to put them "in the zone".

In the medical world, meditation is employed as part of the treatment regime for cancer, chronic pain, heart disease, high blood pressure, asthma, anxiety disorders, depression, neuromuscular disease and insomnia. **Could meditation be more powerful than medication?** There is now ample evidence that meditation delivers profound physical, psychological and emotional benefits. Specifically, meditation has been found to:

- Reduce blood pressure
- Slow breathing and heart rates, thereby counteracting the stress response
- Decrease airway hyper-responsiveness in asthma
- Improve pain management
- Boost immunity to disease and lower the risk of heart attack and cancer
- Elevate the body's production of DHEAS (dehydro-epiandrosterone), a powerful hormone with anti-ageing effects
- Reduce tension, anxiety, depression and fatigue
- Amplify activity in the brain's left prefrontal cortex, which is associated with feeling relaxed and happy
- Raise our sense of self-mastery and inner peace.

Neuroscientists at the Flinders Medical Centre in Adelaide in 2007 found that as people go into a deep, meditative state, their brain rhythms shift into a pattern of focus, thereby activating the NBOM and raising alertness and performance. At Cambridge University, John Teasdale found that meditation reduced the relapse rate in chronically depressed patients by half. In 2006, 11 000 Catholic school students from 31 primary and secondary schools in the Diocese of Townsville in Queensland learnt to meditate for 10 minutes at a time, three times per week, in a world-first project to combat stress and bullying. The results were exemplary: children were calmer and more open to doing schoolwork; teachers reported a reduction in aggression; secondary students requested more meditation sessions prior to exam time; and there wasn't a single negative comment from any parent across all 31 schools. Over 40 studies about meditation for convicted criminals show a drop in recidivism of 30–50 per cent. At the University of Wisconsin at Madison, groups of newly taught meditators and non-meditators were given flu shots, after which they had their blood antibody levels measured. The meditators had more antibodies (a stronger immune response) at both four and eight weeks after the shots. When their brain activity was measured, the meditators also had a shift in activity from the right prefrontal cortex to the left prefrontal cortex, which correlates with higher levels of contentment. The greater the shift in brain activity, the more antibodies they had.

What was I waiting for?

The smorgasbord of meditation options was overwhelming. Evidence suggests that the practice leading to the greatest degree of mental silence confers the greatest benefits. Which would work best for me—Transcendental Meditation (TM), Vipassana Meditation (VM), Sahaja Yoga Meditation (SYM), Inner Body Meditation (IBM), chanting meditation, or one of countless other "brands"?

TM aims to prevent distracting thoughts by repeating a mantra. VM is based on the practice of mindfulness, whereby focused attention on breathing or another physical sensation cultivates mental calmness. SYM teaches the experience of "thoughtless awareness". Inner Body Meditation is about becoming aware of our life force energy.

After rigorous research, I chose the centre which was closest to home, ran classes at convenient times and charged an optional donation. If I experienced inner silence and the promised improvements in my life, I'd stay with it; if not, I'd try a different type of meditation.

I knew after the first session that it was right for me. Out of curiosity, I later tried different types of meditation and found all of them led me to a quiet, peaceful place inside. By the time I'd been meditating for six months, I concluded that *Time's* bubble bath analogy was incomplete. Meditation was really like lying in a bubble bath sipping a cocktail laced with Prozac, painkillers, blood pressure-lowering medications, omega-3s, IQ enhancers and Viagra. Yum!

Sleep

*Sleep is the golden chain that ties health
and our bodies together.*
Thomas Dekker

We don't need scientific research to tell us that when we're tired we get grumpy, run down and mentally sluggish. Nothing is fun, even things that are inherently fun. We get stressed far more easily than when we're rested.

Yet sleep starvation (accumulated sleep deprivation) is an epidemic affecting all generations of Australians. Sleep starvation is associated with depressive symptoms, lowered immunity to disease, impairment of memory functions, poor attention, erosion of decision-making skills, lowered IQ, raised cortisol (stress hormone) levels, lack of empathy, interference with blood glucose regulation and increase in appetite, especially for fat and sugar-rich foods. Our ability to utilise the food we eat drops by about one-third when we fail to get adequate sleep, which further increases our appetite. Chronic sleep deprivation is a significant contributing factor to our current obesity epidemic.

Sleep deficiency also accelerates the ageing process. Six consecutive days of sleep deprivation (averaging four hours of sleep per night) transforms the body chemistry of a healthy 30 year-old into that of a 60 year-old, and it takes almost a week for the body to revert back to normal. Healthy young men who were sleep deprived for one week and then given a flu vaccination had a poorer response to the vaccine (less protection against the flu) than a comparable group of men who were not sleep deprived.

If we learn a new skill during the day, we're much better at it the next day if we get a good night's sleep. Changes in our brains triggered by learning require quiet time to process, to integrate the changes into our existing neuronal circuitry. It's like concrete needing time to set. When we sleep we aren't engaged in conscious thought, but our brains are extremely active. The brain is consolidating learning, establishing lasting memories, organising information and formulating solutions to problems. Students are three times more likely to discover the most efficient way of solving mathematical problems if they have a regular night's sleep between their first and second attempts at finding the solution. To sleep on something is an excellent, scientifically validated idea. Conversely, students, soldiers and solicitors show a 30 per cent drop in cognition and performance after a single night of sleep loss. In the words of Baltasar Gracian, "It is better to sleep on things beforehand than lie awake about them afterwards."

Afternoon Nap

Set aside half an hour every day to do all your worrying;
then take a nap during this period.
Unknown

My father loved his afternoon nap. He said it refreshed him and improved his ability to concentrate.

"And it gives me the energy to cope with all your demands," he pronounced.

For once we agreed—not about my being demanding, but about the benefits of a daily nap. Our brain chemistry favours us taking a nap every afternoon, and this is unrelated to the size or heaviness of our lunch, and regardless of whether or not we had a good night's sleep. We are biologically programmed to have a siesta. Our body temperature drops slightly and we feel transiently sleepy. During this time we are less alert, less productive and more likely to have a car accident.

An afternoon nap improves performance at work and boosts learning at school. Numerous studies on napping have found that it enhances our ability to stay focused, engage in logical reasoning and make complicated decisions. A pilot's performance can be improved by more than 34 per cent after a 26-minute nap. Even a 10-minute nap can improve mood and cognitive function.

Scientists at the Salk Institute for Biological Studies in California found that people who didn't nap showed declining brain performance as the day wore on. In contrast, cognitive function in those who took a nap remained high throughout the day. In a Harvard University study, students were tested four times in one day on their ability to detect subtle changes in an image. Over the course of the first test, the students showed progressive improvement in speed and accuracy. During the second test, the improvements levelled off. The students were then randomly assigned to three groups: napped for 30 minutes, napped for 60 minutes and didn't nap at all. During the third and fourth tests, those who didn't nap scored lower than they had in the second test. Those who napped for 30 minutes showed no drop in their performance, while those who napped for 60 minutes continued to improve their test scores. Neuroscientist Robert Stickgold of Harvard Medical School proposed that, "Napping may protect brain circuits from overuse until those neurons can consolidate what's been learned about a procedure."

How long should a nap be? Some studies suggest 10 minutes is more refreshing than 30 minutes, but anything from a few minutes to one hour has been found to confer benefits. A good night's sleep is anything from six to nine hours, depending on age, gender, hormonal status and individual differences. The ideal length of an afternoon nap may also differ from one person to the next.

Robert Fulghum, in *All I Really Need To Know I Learned in Kindergarten*, wrote, "Think what a better world it would be if we all—the whole world—had cookies and milk about three o'clock every afternoon and then lay down with our blankies for a nap." He is spot on: people from countries in which there is an afternoon siesta tend to have greater longevity and an infectious *joie de vivre*.

Recharging

*Stillness is where creativity and solutions
to problems are found.*
Eckhart Tolle

The boat metaphor for the brain can also be applied to the NBOM. A boat has a battery that enables the boat to run, and this battery needs regular charging. There are three types of battery chargers: bulk chargers, trickle chargers and solar chargers.

A bulk charger recharges a depleted battery. A trickle charger maintains the full capacity of the battery by charging it even while it is discharging. A solar charger converts the sun's rays to low voltage DC electricity, which provides power that can either be used or stored.

The NBOM can be viewed as the brain's battery, and it can be charged in ways analogous to those just described. Bulk charging equates to having a good night's sleep. Trickle charging is equivalent to meditating—we're awake, alert and aware, while at the same time enhancing our capacity to focus and concentrate. The sun is analogous to our attention. We can choose to shine our attention wherever we want, on the past, present or future. If we put our attention on the present, we are energised rather than depleted, no matter how challenging the present situation might be. Paying full attention to what we're doing switches on the NBOM. If we're totally absorbed in dealing with something, it is far less draining than if we divert our attention to concerns about the future or regrets about the past.

Alcohol

Cassio in William Shakespeare's *Othello*

Dad and I have one thing in common: a deficiency of aldehyde dehydrogenase, the liver enzyme needed to break down the toxic elements in alcohol. Put simply, after only a few mouthfuls of alcohol, we throw up.

It's an inherited condition, more frequently seen in people from East Asia, and the more common symptoms following a drink are facial flushing, nasal congestion, headache, tachycardia (rapid heartbeat), palpitations (heart flutters) or nausea, rather than outright vomiting. My father and I have a rather extreme reaction.

When people asked Dad why he was a lifelong teetotaller, he liked to quote Lady Astor, the first woman to sit as a member of parliament in the British House of Commons: "One reason I don't drink is that I want to know when I'm having a good time."

Alcohol intolerance is not a bad thing. Although red wine has received a lot of good press in the last decade, a position statement from the Australian Heart Foundation in 2010 offers sobering advice: red wine is *not* recommended for the prevention or treatment of cardiovascular disease. Instead, we should eat at least two serves of fruit and five serves of vegetables daily, and wash them down with black or green tea.

In relation to the brain, alcohol impairs functioning in the frontal, parietal and temporal lobes, as well as the cerebellum and brain stem. This translates into the signs of acute alcohol intoxication with which most people are familiar: loss of inhibitions, impaired judgement, slower reaction time, slurred speech and lack of muscle coordination. Although brain function reverts to normal when someone sobers up, there are lingering effects and long-term complications of drinking more than two glasses a day for men, and more than one glass a day for women.

There is good news and bad news—please stay with me, even though you might not like what you read! The good news is that alcohol doesn't appear to kill brain cells. The bad news is that it damages dendrites, the branched projections of brain and nerve cells that receive messages from other cells. This results in disruption to communication between brain cells. The good news is that, for the most part, the brain repairs damage to its dendrites. The bad news is that nerve cell structure is changed during repairs and some functions do not return to normal.

The exact mechanisms by which alcohol affects the brain, and the likelihood of reversing the impact of heavy drinking, continue to be studied. Research on animals shows that high doses of alcohol disrupt neurogenesis (the generation of new brain cells), particularly in the hippocampus. Studies on humans show that alcohol also interferes with neurotransmitter release.

What we do know about alcohol and the brain is:

- People who consume more than 14 alcoholic drinks a week— an average of two per day—have significantly smaller brain volumes than people who have less than one drink per day. And there's a direct, dose-dependent relationship: the more we drink, the more we shrink.

- Brain shrinkage is especially extensive in the frontal lobe cortex, the site of higher cognitive functions, and the vulnerability of the frontal lobe to shrinkage increases with age.

- For the equivalent intake of alcohol, women experience more brain shrinkage than men, and women who consume just over one standard drink each day (10 grams of alcohol or 100 millilitres of wine) increase their risk of breast cancer by 24 per cent compared with teetotallers. In 2009 the NSW Cancer Institute attributed 12 per cent of breast cancers to excessive alcohol consumption—which means the cancer was avoidable for more than one in 10 women.

- Although alcohol acts as a sedative in the acute intoxication stage, it diminishes the quality of sleep and produces longer and more severe episodes of hypoxia (oxygen deprivation) in people with sleep apnoea.

- The most significant factor determining the extent of alcohol-induced brain impairment is the maximum amount consumed at any one time and the frequency with which we consume such amounts. Regular binge drinking is the worst thing we can do for our brains.

- At a conservative estimate, long-term alcohol abuse accounts for 4 per cent of cases of dementia in Western countries.

- We perform better in anything that requires sharp mental acuity if we abstain from alcohol for 24 hours prior to the event.

The only thing that sobers us up is time. Contrary to common opinion, coffee and caffeine products do *not* shorten the time it takes to sober up. The liver is responsible for eliminating alcohol and other toxins from the bloodstream, and coffee does not affect the rate at which this occurs. Coffee may make you feel more awake, but alertness doesn't equate to sobriety. In fact, hot liquids have been shown to speed up the rate at which alcohol is absorbed from the stomach into the bloodstream, so drinking coffee with alcohol can result in getting drunk even more quickly.

It has been wisely noted: "If you know someone who tries to drown their sorrows, you might want to tell them that sorrows know how to swim."

Arsenic

Food, one assumes, provides nourishment, but Americans eat it fully aware that small amounts of poison have been added to improve its appearance and delay its putrefaction.
John Cage

"Where's the Coca-Cola?" Dad called out.

"I used it to clean the mould off the laundry windowsill," I replied.

"You *what*?" he asked incredulously.

"Coca-Cola is an excellent cleaning agent. You spill it on for about 30 seconds and then rinse it off. If you leave it too long, it'll start to erode the wood."

"You're nuts. So what is there for me to drink?"

"Filtered water. It's in the fridge."

"I'm going to the shops to get some soft drinks."

"Soft drinks shouldn't be consumed by humans. I know a large percentage of the population drink them, but that's because they don't realise just how damaging they are to the body, brain, mood and energy levels. I think drinking soft drinks is akin to ingesting arsenic: it doesn't kill you straightaway but over time it wreaks havoc throughout the body."

"Arsenic has been used medicinally for centuries, especially in China," my father flatly replied. "It was used to treat syphilis before Fleming discovered penicillin."

"Humans engaged in a lot of destructive habits over the centuries, before they realised how harmful they were," I countered. "Victorian era women applied a mixture containing arsenic to their skin in an attempt to combat wrinkles. Now we know better. Smoking is another example—cigarette companies argued for decades that cigarettes weren't harmful. Soft drinks should carry the same warnings as cigarettes."

"Have you ever come across the concept of moderation? One soft drink isn't going to do anyone any harm."

"Yes, it is. A 375 millilitre can of Coca-Cola has more than 10 teaspoons of sugar, 45 milligrams of caffeine, 150 calories and the acidity of vinegar, with no nutritional value apart from the energy in the calories, which most people can do without. Soft drinks are up there as major contributors to obesity, diabetes, mood swings, hyperactivity and, paradoxically, lethargy.

"**Don't damage the boat**. If you want to improve your memory and mental function, give up the soft drinks. They lead to sluggish thinking. Fizzy drinks make fuzzy brains. Research conducted in 2003 demonstrated that children who consumed soft drinks and sugary snacks for breakfast performed at the level of a mentally compromised 70 year-old in tests of memory and attention."

"I'm already a mentally compromised 70 year-old."

"I wonder if that has anything to do with the fact that you've been drinking soft drinks every day for 60 years?"

"OK, I'll buy diet lemon squash."

"Sorry. A US study of more than 9 500 adults found that drinking diet soft drinks was also associated with an increased risk of metabolic syndrome (a combination of disorders that increases the risk of developing cardiovascular disease and diabetes). After the nine-year research period, almost 40 per cent of participants had developed three or more indicators of metabolic syndrome."

"How is that possible if there's no sugar in them?"

"Possibly because diet soft drinks stimulate the appetite and give you an acquired taste for high sweetness. They can even give you tooth decay, especially when you have low levels of saliva, which happens when you're thirsty."

Dad scowled.

"Look," I said, "do you really want to be drinking a strange mixture of phosphorous, phosphoric acid, caffeine, sodium, artificial colouring, flavouring, preservatives and nutrient-depleting additives?"

"You are *so* hard to live with," Dad concluded. "If anyone is ever mad enough to ask for your hand in marriage, I'm going to sit him down with a long list of warnings."

Walnuts

Food is an important part of a balanced diet.
Fran Lebowitz

"What's *this*?" Dad was looking at the handful of walnuts and half-punnet of blueberries I'd put out with his morning medications.

"It's two more medicines for you: walnuts for the omega-3 fatty acids and blueberries because they promote cell growth in the hippocampus. Feeding blueberry extract to older rats improves their spatial memory and their ability to navigate through a maze. **Feed your brain the finest.**"

"Why are omega-3s supposed to be so good for your brain?" My father was in one of his inquisitive moods.

"Because 60 per cent of your brain composition is structural fat, primarily omega-3 polyunsaturated fatty acids. The three most nutritionally important omega-3 fatty acids are alpha-linolenic acid (ALA), eicosapentaenoic acid (EPA) and docosahexaenoic acid (DHA). The body can convert ALA into EPA and DHA, but it can only get ALA from your diet."

"And walnuts are a source of ALA?" He was still playing with them, not eating them.

"Yes. Walnuts along with linseeds and linseed oil (also known as flaxseed oil), soy beans and dark green, leafy vegetables, like spinach."

"I'll take the walnuts."

"The richest sources of EPA and DHA are cold water, deep sea fish, such as salmon, sardines, cod, herring, mackerel, trevally, snapper and tuna. Epidemiological studies suggest that eating fish several times a week is associated with a reduced risk of developing depression and Alzheimer's Disease, but if everyone in the world ate fish more than once a week it would be an environmental disaster. Seventy-five per cent of the world's fish supply is fully or partially over-exploited already.

"And while we're on the subject, it's just as important to reduce your intake of omega-6s as it is to increase your intake of omega-3s. Although omega-6 fatty acids are also essential for human health, the required ratio of omega-6 to omega-3 fatty acids is 2–4 times more omega-6s than omega-3s. But the typical Australian and American diets consist of *10–20* times more omega-6s than omega-3s. Did you get that? We're eating *10* times more omega-6s than we need, and this imbalance is implicated in heart disease, diabetes, dementia and a host of other inflammatory conditions."

"So what do I have to give up now?"

"You'll be very happy to know that you don't have to give up eating any foods. You just need to give up junk food, which of course isn't food, it's junk. Junk for the body and junk for the brain."

"And what are you calling junk food?"

"Junk food is high sugar-, high salt- and high unhealthy fat-containing processed food, that usually has a long list of additives, preservatives, artificial colourings and nefarious ingredients represented by numbers. It includes commercial biscuits, packaged cakes, pastries, sugary breakfast cereals, chips, salty snacks, chocolate bars, boxed meals and frozen dinners. A rule of thumb: if your grandmother wouldn't recognise it as food, it probably isn't."

My father rolled his eyes.

"Dad, I'm not trying to make your life miserable; I'm trying to tell you that what you eat affects the chemicals in your brain, which affects your mood and your mental processes. How could it not? Everything we eat leaves its mark on us. Everything we eat is incorporated into our body and our brain. Junk food is pollution in our body. Junk food leads to general slowing of all brain functions and contributes to poor learning, mood swings and mental and physical fatigue. You'll get a new lease on life when you start eating *real* food. It's just like putting the right fuel in a motor—performance improves immeasurably."

He sighed his irritating sigh. "So what's the best fuel for my brain?"

"Scientists are still trying to figure it out but it looks like eating healthy fats—that means omega-3 fatty acids, monounsaturated fats like olive oil, and saturated fats like coconut oil and butter— plus moderate amounts of protein and plenty of non-starchy vegetables, is the best way to go.

"Why does the brain need proteins?"

"Proteins get broken down into amino acids, which are used to make neurotransmitters. Neurotransmitters are chemical messengers that transmit signals between nerve cells. Trust me— you're getting enough protein in your diet. Most people in the Developed World eat more protein than they need."

"Which is how much?"

"Your protein requirements depend on your body weight and level of physical activity. A rough guide is approximately 0.8 grams of protein per kilogram of body weight per day. So for you, weighing in at 70kg, it means you need 56 grams of protein a day. If you sit around playing Sudoku from morning till night, you need less protein. If you come to the gym with me every day, you can eat more protein—up to 1.5 grams per kilogram. That would take it up to 105 grams a day for you."

"You're wicked."

My heart went out to Dad. Was I being too hard on him? Was I expecting too much? Was my reliance on science preventing me from seeing that he needed reassurance and autonomy more than he needed omega-3s and blueberries? I was terrified of losing him to dementia before I had the opportunity of finding him. I wanted his latter years to be the best they could be—but what constitutes "the best they could be"? Was I feeding his brain at the expense of soothing his soul? Was I behaving like a well-meaning yet misguided parent, blinded by her own agenda? I was beginning to question my approach. I had no doubt about the brain-boosting benefits of everything I asked him to do, but maybe I was neglecting his emotional needs in the process. Allowing him to eat junk food would feel like elder abuse to me, but it might be comforting to him. Perhaps I needed to listen more and talk less.

Attitude

*The meaning we attribute to old age shapes the very meaning of
our entire cycle of human life.*
Simone de Beauvoir

Our attitude to ageing has a measurable effect on our longevity.
In a 2002 research paper, Becca Levy recorded that people with
more positive perceptions of ageing lived an average of seven-
and-a-half years longer than people who felt negatively about
ageing. This was after gender, socioeconomic status, loneliness
and overall health were taken into account. In fact, *the effect of
a positive attitude on survival was greater than the effect of a healthy
lifestyle!* Having low blood pressure, normal cholesterol levels
and never smoking each added around four extra years to life—
only half of what a life-affirming, optimistic outlook gives!

What's more, the effects of encouraging statements were found
to be immediate as well as long term. Elderly people exposed to
positive and constructive messages about ageing immediately
before a series of memory tests performed better than individuals
told or shown something negative in relation to ageing. Even just
having sanguine words flashed in front of them momentarily,
without the individual being consciously aware of it, led to
higher scores.

In another landmark study, a team of psychologists from the
University of Kentucky discovered that optimism in general
is associated with a longer lifespan. The researchers studied
autobiographies penned by a congregation of 180 Catholic nuns
on 22 September 1930. On this day, the mother superior had
asked all the sisters in her order, whose average age was 22, to
write a brief autobiography. More than 70 years later, the letters
were carefully scrutinised for words suggesting positive and
negative emotions. Positive words included happiness, joy, love,

hope, gratitude and contentment; negative words were sadness, fear, confusion, disappointment and shame. The researchers found that nuns who expressed more positive emotions in their autobiographies lived significantly longer—in some instances by 10 years—than those expressing fewer positive emotions. For every 1 per cent increase in the number of sentences with positive emotion, the researchers found a 1.4 per cent decrease in the women's mortality rate. Of the nuns who wrote the most positive sentences, less than a quarter (24 per cent) had died. Of those who wrote the least number of positive sentences, more than half (54 per cent) had died. The average age at death for the least positive nuns was 86 years and for the happiest it was 93.5 years. In either case, nuns are laughing all the way to heaven.

I decided to introduce display cards to our house. I typed up a list of positive statements of particular relevance for Dad and put them up around the house, several in every room. Some were quotes from "successful agers", some were uplifting medical facts about ageing, and some would hopefully bring a smile to his face. I decided it didn't matter whether he consciously noticed them or not; such was the power of subliminal advertising. The list of affirmations was:

We make 5 000 new brain cells every day of our lives.

Do what you can with what you have, where you are. Theodore Roosevelt

Radical improvements in cognitive functioning are possible until the day we die.

The way I see it, if you want the rainbow, you gotta put up with the rain. Dolly Parton

Every year of life adds another book to our internal library of resources.

Ageing enables us to turn wounds into wisdom.

Nature, time and patience are the three great physicians.
Chinese proverb

When you tell the truth, you never have to worry about a lousy memory.

The world unwraps itself to us, again and again, as soon as we're ready to see it anew. Fiyero in Wicked

One of the wonders of life is just that—the wonder of life.
Bill Copeland

Age is an issue of mind over matter. If you don't mind, it doesn't matter. Mark Twain

Do your little bit of good where you are; it's those little bits of good put together that overwhelm the world. Archbishop Desmond Tutu

Ageing is a funny thing. Treasured in a tree, in wine, in furniture, in everything, but me.

To live is so startling it leaves little time for anything else.
Emily Dickinson

Doing the best at this moment puts us in the best place for the next moment. Oprah Winfrey

At 20 we worry about what others think of us; at 40 we don't care about what others think of us; at 60 we discover they haven't been thinking about us at all.

The time is always right to do what is right. Martin Luther King, Jr

I intend to live forever. Or die trying. Groucho Marx

Gratitude

God gave you a gift of 86 400 seconds today.
Have you used one to say, 'Thank you'?
William A. Ward

"Dad, I have a present for you."

"Oh no," he complained, "your presents always mean work."

I handed my father a brightly wrapped, rectangular package that he duly opened.

"It's a notebook. What am I supposed to take notes on?" he asked.

"It's your Gratitude Journal," I announced. "At the end of every day, you write down what you're grateful for. Anything that comes to mind—things that happened during the day or things that you're generally thankful for. And the next morning, you read what you wrote the night before. Let's practise together right now." My father gave me his familiar weary look. "Tell me five things you're thankful for," I encouraged.

"I can't think of anything."

"OK then, I'll start," I offered. "I'm grateful that I have so many wonderful friends. Your turn."

Dad thought for a moment. "I'm grateful that Marko is my friend." I turned away so he wouldn't see me scowl.

"I'm grateful that I love my work," I continued. "I regard my work as play."

"I'm grateful that I've retired from work," he said.

I shook my head. Why were things never as straightforward as I anticipated them to be?

"I'm grateful that I'm fit and healthy."

"I'm grateful that *you're* fit and healthy."

"Oh stop it! You have to come up with your own ideas. What's something in your life that you really appreciate?"

"I am deeply appreciative that you're in good health," he replied, "otherwise you wouldn't be able to look after me."

"I'm appreciative that you're appreciative. Now, how about something relating to yourself that you appreciate?"

My father was silent for a long time. "I'm grateful that I'm still capable of going to the gym with you, even if sometimes I'd rather stay home."

"Fantastic! Now you've got the hang of it. Tell me more."

For the first few weeks, extracting statements of gratitude from Dad was akin to extracting splinters. However, with practice, he got onto a "gratitude wavelength" and counting his blessings ceased to be arduous.

Regularly reflecting on things that we're grateful for creates a perceptual filter through which to view life. Gratitude becomes the context in which we relate to the world, and we begin to notice more things to be grateful for. We snap out of taking things for granted and become aware of the wonder of life. We see the sun peeping from behind the clouds, even on an overcast day. In the same way that asking "how" questions mobilises the subconscious mind to find solutions to problems, expressing gratitude opens the door to a new way of seeing the world. We begin to see what we have, rather than what we don't have, and we become a magnet for experiences that support feeling thankful. In the words of Jacqueline Winspear, "Grace isn't a little prayer you chant before receiving a meal. It's a way to live."

At the University of California, psychologist Robert Emmons found that gratitude exercises improved physical health, raised energy levels, increased people's overall satisfaction with life and even reduced pain and fatigue in patients with neuromuscular disease. People who elaborated more, and had a wider span of things they were grateful for, experienced the greatest benefits. In a study of adolescents, asking them to count blessings was associated with enhanced optimism, mood and satisfaction with school, even though nothing in their external circumstances had changed.

Practising gratitude can take many forms. It can mean ordering a coffee with genuine thanks; sending a thank you card; telling someone how much we appreciate them; or keeping a gratitude journal. Gratitude exercises were a way of reminding my father that there was still joy to be found in life. I wanted him to relive positive feelings as often as possible, to reinforce them and make them a habit. We are at our most suggestible and impressionable just before sleep and in the first few minutes of waking. What he thought about, and what I said to him first thing in the morning and last thing before sleep, had the greatest impact on his subconscious mind and his outlook on life.

The first change I observed in Dad after starting his gratitude journal was the way he greeted me in the morning. The pattern since my mother had died was for me to open with, "Good morning, Dad". My father would respond, "Is it? I hadn't noticed."

I considered it a major victory when he began replying, "Good morning".

Three Strikes

*The only people with whom you should try to get even
are those who have helped you.*
John E. Southard

"I've thought of something you can be grateful for," my father offered one evening. "You can be grateful to me for the longevity of your current relationship."

"What?!"

Dan and I were seeing less of each other now that we lived a 30-minute drive apart, as opposed to when we'd lived a 90-minute flight apart, and the reason was none other than my newly acquired filial responsibilities.

"Anyone you spend a substantial amount of time with ends up disappearing quick smart," Dad said, "and I don't blame them. Now that you have me to prevent you from seeing much of Dan, the man has a chance of remaining happily deluded for a lot longer."

"Gee, thanks." I wasn't going to fall into the trap of asking what Dan was purportedly deluded about.

"Do you ever hear from your ex-boyfriend, Greg? He was lucky to get out alive."

This was sadly true. Despite warning Greg on our first date that I might be good at maths and science, but I was clueless when it came to long-term relationships, he was ready to move in within a month. But after almost putting him in hospital on three occasions within six months, he finally realised he'd better go home—for good.

Incident #1: I was calmly brushing my hair in the bathroom before going to bed. I had tipped my head forward, so my view of anything above me was obscured. Unbeknown to me, Greg entered the bathroom and leant over me just as I swung my head back up. CRUNCH!—the sound of shattering bone and twisted cartilage, accompanied by blood spurting across the mirror. Greg lay in agony at my feet, holding his nose and covering his left eye. It didn't look good. I dragged him onto a towel and emptied a bucket of ice onto his face. More groans. Half an hour later, I pried his hands away to reveal a swollen, crimson, disfigured mess. His nose resembled an overripe eggplant and his eye was buried in a puffed up, spongy socket. It was not a comfortable night for either of us. I felt terrible for not only inflicting such grievous bodily harm but for shamefully muttering under my breath, "How many times do I need to tell you—I need more space!"

Incident #2: In a doorway of my Brisbane apartment I'd installed a removable chin-up bar, which I sometimes forgot to remove. This posed no problems if you were the same height as I was. But if you were considerably taller (which Greg was), and if you were in a hurry (which Greg was), you could do considerable damage to your forehead (which Greg did).

Incident #3: My electric blanket had stopped working. Greg, being a "real man" with a mathematical-plus-handyman brain, offered to fix it. I gave him my toolkit and left him alone, while I went to water the plants on the balcony. As I walked past, I dripped some water where he was working—BANG! Greg somersaulted past me, leaving a black hole where the on/off switch had once been.

Oops.

Imagination

Imagination is more important than knowledge. For knowledge is limited to all we now know and understand, while imagination embraces the entire world, and all there ever will be to know and understand.
Albert Einstein

Dad always forgot to take his morning and evening medications. This wasn't a problem when we ate breakfast and dinner together because I'd remind him and watch him taking them. However, if I wasn't there, he never remembered. Even when I rang and told him, "As soon as you hang up, go and take your medications" he would forget. Often I insisted that he take his medications while I waited on the phone, but he considered this to be ridiculous and he frequently refused.

I thought that I could solve the problem by writing "Take your medications after you eat this" on the same piece of paper as I'd written "Dad's dinner", but he threw out the piece of paper along with the gladwrap and by the end of the meal he'd forgotten again. Even writing "Take your medications after dinner" on the fridge whiteboard didn't work. We'd gone past the point where he deliberately omitted taking his medications. I'd convinced him that stopping his tablets would only make him more miserable and breathless, without necessarily hastening his trip to the grave. So he no longer objected to his medications—he just genuinely forgot to take them. Finally, I tried a completely different tactic.

In a study by Liu and Park published in 2004, older people needing to check their blood sugar levels were 50 per cent more likely to remember to do so if they spent three minutes every morning visualising themselves performing the task. What would happen if I asked Dad to visualise himself eating and then taking his medications?

"You're the one losing her mind," he responded when I first suggested it. Part of the problem was that he didn't remember that he didn't remember. "Will you leave me in peace if I go along with this?" he asked. I nodded. "OK," he said unenthusiastically.

"Close your eyes and imagine seeing yourself eating the chicken vegetable soup," I began. "Do you have a picture of it in your mind? … Imagine how it smells and tastes … Imagine the warm liquid passing down your throat … Yum. See yourself finishing the last spoonful of soup and reaching for your blue pillbox … Pull down the thin, plastic window for Saturday's pills. Hear the click as the plastic hits the base. Take the box in your left hand and tip it upside down, so the tablets fall into your right hand … Pick up a glass of water …"

"Lemonade!"

"We don't have lemonade. Sorry. Put the tablets in your mouth and wash them down with the refreshing water. Close the window of your pillbox and put the box back in its place on the shelf. Now, open your eyes … How was that?"

"Riveting. Who needs TV?" I paid no attention to his sarcasm.

"Were you able to picture the whole thing in your mind?" I quizzed.

"As I said, just like watching TV. Tell me, how is this going to help me remember to take my medications?"

"When you use your imagination, you engage a less sophisticated, automatic part of your brain's memory machinery, one that is more robust than other parts of our memory. So even if some parts of your memory are declining, you're likely to remember things that you *imagine* more readily than things that you actually *do*. Your imagination creates what scientists call a neural footprint of what you want to remember."

"Right."

I smiled. "Enjoy your dinner and I'll see you in a few hours." By 9 pm I couldn't hold back; I had to ring.

"How was dinner? Did you take your medications?"

"Of course."

"Really?"

"You sound surprised."

"Can you go and check your pillbox, just to be sure?"

"You're a real nuisance, do you know that?"

"Yes, I do, you tell me often. Just humour me." He went and checked.

"What day is it today?"

"Saturday."

"Yes, the box is empty under Saturday."

I was so excited! Thereafter, I made certain that Dad visualised himself taking his medications every morning and before every excursion I made out of the house. He protested but nonetheless humoured me. It worked 100 per cent of the time.

Perfect Practice

*Logic will get you from A to B. Imagination will take you
everywhere ... It is the preview of life's coming attractions.*
Albert Einstein

Phenomenal as it is, the brain can't tell the difference between what's real and what's imagined. The same neurons fire and the same parts of the brain light up, whether we're *looking* at a cat or whether we have our eyes closed and are *imagining* a cat, or whether we're *playing* the piano or *imagining* ourselves playing the piano. Why is this important? Because it means our thoughts have the power to switch on brain cell activity.

In *The Brain That Changes Itself*, Norman Doidge describes two experiments that demonstrate that **mental practice helps make perfect**. In the first experiment, two groups of people with no previous experience were taught to play the piano. One group did standard, real-life piano practice. The other group imagined their fingers pressing the correct keys and imagined hearing the music—they did no physical practice whatsoever, never touching a keyboard. After three days, both groups played with the same accuracy. After five days, the real-life practice group was slightly better than the mental practice group. However, after a single, two-hour session in which they actually played the piece, the mental students were as good as the real-life students. In the second experiment, researchers found that purely imagining exercising a finger muscle resulted in a 22 per cent increase in the strength of that muscle, compared with a 30 per cent increase in strength if the muscle was physically exercised.

Every time we have a thought, we fire an electrical signal through a neural pathway. Each signal thickens the myelin sheath that surrounds the nerve fibre. The thicker the sheath, the more efficient the signal and the more proficient we are at the skill in question. The more vividly we're able to imagine what it is we want to achieve, the stronger the signal we send to our brains. The more senses and emotions we engage while we're mentally practising, the more parts of the brain we recruit. And the more of the brain we employ, the more effective our mental practice. Persistence is paramount. Just as physical practice leads to greater skill, the more mental practice we do, the better we get. One daydreaming session won't cut it.

The implications of this are enormously exciting and widespread. It means that patients who have injuries that render them bedridden can still engage in mental exercise to help maintain muscle strength. People who have injured limbs can exercise them mentally before they're physically capable of doing so, and thereby greatly speed up healing. Equally exciting is the application of mental practice to achieving goals such as weight loss, overcoming phobias and countless other psychological issues.

Athletes, chess players and performers already use mental practice. In another experiment, it was *even more* effective than physical practice when it came to shooting hoops in basketball. In this particular scenario, there were three groups: one group practised on the court, one group imagined playing, and the third group did no practice whatsoever, physical or mental. After three weeks, the group that practised on the court were the fittest, but the group that only imagined shooting hoops actually scored the highest percentage of shots. The reason postulated for this is that the players who engaged in mental practice engaged in *perfect* practice—they never saw themselves missing. The group physically on the court missed shots, so they weren't always strengthening the correct neural pathways. *Perfect* practice is what makes perfect.

Mental practice ties in with "minding our language" and having a "can do" attitude. Whenever we label ourselves as incompetent, we strengthen a negative mental image of ourselves and thereby "practise" under-performing in the real world. Whenever Dad labelled himself as old, tired or incapable, I asked him to imagine himself as being the opposite. Given that he remembered what he imagined more easily than what he actually did, this was a powerful way of improving his self-confidence.

Part V
Changing *My* Mind

You must be the change you want to see in the world.

Mahatma Gandhi

Dry-Cleaning

*The search for happiness is one of the chief sources
of unhappiness.*
Eric Hoffer

Dan and I hadn't been on a date without Dad for over a month. But tonight was the night. It was a crisp, blustery winter evening and I was about to slip into a slinky, snug, seductive, black coat, which my father had brought back from dry-cleaning that morning. The coat looked pristine, feminine and alluring—the way I would feel while wearing it.

As I excitedly slipped the coat on, there was a loud snap, crackle and pop, and before I could fathom what was happening, the coat seemed to disintegrate. It just fell to pieces and embedded itself into the sleeve of my evening dress. I couldn't believe it. When I tried to pull off the coat, more destruction took place and before I knew it, I had a pile of black fluff and shredded, plastic-like material all over the carpet. I tried shaking the black, sticky fibres from my dress, but the only way to remove them was to hand-pluck each shred off. My father walked in just as I was ready to howl.

"What have you done to that lovely dress?" he asked.

"I haven't done anything! My coat has imploded and implanted itself in my outfit."

"You can't go out looking like that," he affirmed the obvious.

I stormed into my room and hurriedly rummaged around for something else to wear. I ended up grabbing a coat of my mother's, which was three sizes too big and anything but alluring. I saw the faintest flicker of a raised eyebrow when Dan greeted me, but he refrained from comment. I spent the first half-hour of our date ranting about the disaster that had just befallen me. Dad kindly spent half the evening vacuuming the remains of the coat from the carpet.

The following morning, when I'd regained my composure, I checked the coat's label. It read "Dry-Clean Only", so I rang the dry-cleaners. They insisted they'd done nothing wrong and I should contact the store where I'd bought the coat. I rang the store. They insisted there was nothing wrong with the coat, and obviously the dry-cleaners can't have known what they were doing. After a week of to-ing and fro-ing, I finally received a full refund from the store, with a request to take my future coat-buying business elsewhere.

A fortnight later, I sent Dad to a different dry-cleaner with a black dress to get it cleaned for a formal dinner I was attending. The dress had a beautiful swirl of black beads sewn across the front bodice. I left the dress in the dry-cleaner's plastic until it was time to put it on, but then one look in the mirror told me something was drastically wrong. The beads had disappeared and in their place were uneven, fraying threads, like weeds in a garden. I called my father into the room.

"Did the dry-cleaner tell you anything when you went to pick up the dress?"

"No."

"Did she give you a little bag of beads, by any chance?"

"No."

"So where have all the beads from my dress disappeared to?"

"The dry-cleaning solvent probably dissolved them," Dad replied matter-of-factly.

"I see. You didn't think to mention this might happen when I gave you the dress to take to the dry-cleaners?"

"You're always telling me you know what you're doing," he stated. "How am I supposed to know when you're kidding yourself?"

I took a long, deep, conscious breath in and then slowly exhaled. Once again, I hurriedly rummaged around for something else to wear.

The following morning, when I'd regained my composure, I checked the label on the dress. It read "Dry-Clean Only", so I rang the dry-cleaners. They insisted they'd done nothing wrong and I should contact the store where I'd bought the dress. I rang the store. They insisted there was nothing wrong with the dress or the beads, and obviously the dry-cleaners can't have known what they were doing. After a week of to-ing and fro-ing, and no refund forthcoming, dad, daughter and dress turned up at the dry-cleaners.

"Good morning", I began. "I had this dress dry-cleaned a week ago and when I was about to wear it, I noticed that all the beads on the front bodice had come off. You can see the threads where they were attached. Is it you I've been speaking to on the phone about this?"

"I knew it was going to be one of those days," scowled the woman behind the counter. "No, it isn't me you've been speaking to; I've been on holidays for the last fortnight. I wasn't supposed to be back at work until tomorrow, but Margaret called in sick at the last minute, so I had to drop everything and race in here."

"I see," I said cautiously. "Well, it appears the solvent has dissolved the beads."

"Yes, it happens quite frequently," continued the scowler. "Dresses like this shouldn't be dry-cleaned."

"But the label says 'Dry-Clean Only'."

"It shouldn't." There was silence. I tried to remain curious and uncritical.

"Regardless of whether the label should or shouldn't recommend dry-cleaning," I ventured, "the dress has been dry-cleaned and the outcome is an unwearable garment. I see that you also arrange tailoring and alterations. Perhaps you'd be able to replace the missing beads for me?"

The scowl widened. "If *I'd* been here when you'd first brought the dress in, I'd have told you to take it home and hand wash it. There's no reason this material couldn't be washed in water."

"Thank you, I'll certainly do that in future. But with the state the dress is in now, it won't be washed again because it won't be worn again. Do you think you could contact your menders and have them restore this to a condition where I'll be able to take your sound advice?"

The scowl returned to its previous diameter. "Leave the dress and ring mid next week."

Five phone calls and three weeks later, I had a newly beaded dress—it had involved buying the beads myself, but at least the dress was as good as new. And the incident created a job for my father: to find yet another local dry-cleaner.

Titanium

Self-confidence is the memory of success.
Unknown

Dad's glasses needed new lenses, so I took him to an optometrist. When the friendly young woman finished examining his eyes, he handed her his 30 year-old titanium frames. She smiled brightly and informed him that under his health insurance policy, he could receive new frames with lenses for only $20, whereas to fit new lenses into his existing frames would cost $138.50.

"Let's look around the store for some new frames," I proposed.

"No, I don't want new frames. None of them will be as good as the ones I already have," he asserted.

"Why don't we take a look anyway," I coaxed. "There have been a lot of advances in the last 30 years."

"I like my frames precisely because they're 30 years old," he insisted. "Doesn't that speak for itself? Nothing is made to last any more. I don't want some newfangled thing that will break in three months."

"Our frames should last for years, unless you drop them or someone steps on them," the optometrist reassured.

"And $20 is practically giving them away," I continued the campaign.

"Nothing you have comes close to my frames," my father claimed. He pushed his glasses towards the optometrist for her to inspect. "They're classy, they're Longines and they're made of pure titanium. Titanium was named after the Titans in Greek mythology. It has the highest strength-to-weight ratio of any metal and is corrosion-resistant. You could throw me into the ocean or push me into a swimming pool and my glasses would remain completely intact because neither sea water nor chlorine can corrode them. Titanium is used in aircraft and spacecraft—that's how indestructible it is. The Soviet Union even made submarines out of titanium."

The optometrist and I exchanged helpless glances while Dad continued.

"We have two fridges at home. One of them we bought within the first year of arriving in Australia, which makes it 38 years old. It's still in perfect working order. Five years ago we bought a second fridge and it's already been repaired three times. I will not have the same thing happen to my glasses. Please fit the new lenses into the original frames."

The optometrist looked pleadingly from me to my father, waiting for a consensus. I didn't feel like giving away $118 for what I considered to be no valid reason.

"Why don't we give it a go with some new frames," I suggested, "and if you're not happy with them, we can always come back and have the lenses fitted into your old frames. No-one's asking you to part with your old frames."

"I don't like any of the new frames. I look much better in the titanium," he insisted.

Here was a man who ordinarily didn't care about anything but was suddenly adamant about a pair of glasses. I opened my mouth with another objection, when I became aware of an uneasy feeling in my stomach. All his life, Dad had given in to Mum. I'd never seen him exert his autonomy. When I'd questioned him about it, he'd said it was futile arguing with my mother because she was relentless—she would always get her way in the end. So why waste time, energy and emotion arguing when it never changed the outcome?

In psychology-speak, Dad was describing "learned helplessness". If a person sees that no matter what he does or how hard he tries, he can't influence an outcome, he'll stop trying and "learn" that he's helpless. When he is then presented with a challenge that he could easily overcome, he doesn't even make an attempt because he has lost faith in his own efficacy. The fact that my father cared about something—anything at all—was a huge step forward. The fact that he was also being assertive was amazing progress. I wanted him to become more self-reliant and to feel that his opinion mattered.

"All right," I agreed. "Please fit the new lenses into the old frames."

"It will be more economical in the long run," Dad reaffirmed.

Packing: Take 2

One's destination is never a place, but a new way
of seeing things.
Henry Miller

Dad and I were going to Tangalooma Resort on Moreton Island, the third largest sand island in the world, located an hour's boat trip from Brisbane. I was running a workshop called **Boost Your Brain and Get Ahead**. My client had not only offered to pay for my father to accompany me, but to have the experience of hand-feeding the wild dolphins that visited Tangalooma jetty each night.

I was thrilled—until it came to the packing. I remembered the heart-wrenching experience of a month ago and considered packing my father's suitcase without his input. It would certainly be the most expedient option but it would also be admitting defeat. My goal was to make Dad more self-reliant, which meant finding a way of making the job achievable for him. What if the packing list I typed was more specific than last time? And what if I then disappeared from the house for an hour? Left to his own devices, what would he do?

I handed my father what looked like an essay, and we sat down and went through it together. I answered his questions and he said he was up to the task. I asked him to tick off each item after he'd put it in the bag, so he'd keep track of where he was up to. Then I went for a jog—at least I would be pumped full of endorphins when I got back.

I had imagined many possible scenarios on my return, but nothing like the spectacle that greeted me. As soon as I opened the front door, I was saluted by a burst of colourful garments, reminiscent of a Mardi Gras parade. Every painting, wood-carving and tapestry in our hallway had a garish, floral shirt draped over it. My client intended to hold a loud shirt competition and judging from the display in front of me, Dad was a sure winner. The TV was obscured by shoes, socks and underwear; the couch was covered with trousers and shorts; every door handle served as a hat hook; and the table lamp flaunted a pair of bathers. But my father's suitcase was empty.

Dad had retired to his room to read *Harry Potter and the Goblet of Fire*. There was a note on the kitchen table: "I couldn't be sure what you wanted me to pack, so I've laid out all the variables for you to make your selection."

I laughed and laughed and laughed and ...

Calendar

To be yourself in a world that is constantly trying to make you something else is the greatest accomplishment.
Ralph Waldo Emerson

"It's present time again," I smiled, as I handed Dad a large, brown paper bag.

"Oh no! Enough of your presents!" he backed away.

"This one is really fun," I encouraged.

"You have a warped sense of fun. Whenever you say something is fun, it fills me with dread."

I placed the bag in his hands. He sat down in resignation and looked inside.

"A calendar?" he queried. "What's this about?"

"This calendar is your personal assistant. It's your appointment and job reminder system and your record of daily events. You keep telling me you're becoming forgetful and that you never know what's in store for the week. Now you'll know exactly what's happening a month at a time because this is the first thing you'll see every morning and the last thing you'll check every night. Whenever we make an appointment to see someone or do something, write it on the calendar. Whenever I ask you to do something on a particular day, write it on the calendar. At the end of every day, write up everything you did that wasn't planned ahead. Then put a red line through the day, so you'll know what day it is the next day. And it'll be your job to tell me the day and the date every morning. I'm sticking the calendar at one end of the kitchen table, so it'll stay there permanently. At the end of each month we'll replace it with the next month and keep the completed months in this folder, so you can look back on what you've done at any time."

"And that's your idea of fun?"

"Absolutely! It's fun feeling organised and looking back at what you've accomplished."

"But I'm not exactly accomplishing things."

"Of course you are. Keeping on top of your health is accomplishing something. Going to the gym is accomplishing something. Giving a lonely person a few hours of social stimulation is definitely accomplishing something. Helping someone move house is accomplishing something. You're becoming a regular neighbourhood helping hand. And a calendar is essential to stay on top of when you need to be somewhere. Then you won't have to rely on me to tell you all the time."

For once, Dad approached what I suggested with a degree of enthusiasm. For the first few weeks I regularly repeated the instructions I'd given him about the calendar, and I sat with him as he wrote his entries. With time, he took ownership of the calendar and it became his morning and evening ritual. It transformed both our lives. My father had a new-found confidence and the first hint of a sense of purpose.

Nothing in his life had changed except his feeling of control over it.

Excitement

Don't ask what the world needs. Ask what makes you come alive and go do it. Because what the world needs is people who have come alive.
Howard Thurman

"I can give you all the omega-3s and blueberries you like, but you're still missing the most powerful brain fuel of all," I declared.

"And what's that?" my father asked.

"Excitement! Passion! Enthusiasm for life! Enthusiasm for *anything*. I know that's a tough ask and I know you miss Mum and I know that losing her is still an overwhelming shock, but you weren't bursting with enthusiasm for anything while Mum was alive either. That's what saddens me the most: absolutely nothing arouses your interest. Being interested in things, apart from enhancing your enjoyment of life, is essential for your brain to remain sharp. Staying curious about the world and continuing to set goals, big or small, is what keeps your spirit, your brain and your body alive. If you put demands on your brain to keep learning, exploring and engaging with life, your brain will deliver because that's what it's designed to do. We're never too old to dream and go for it. Whether we realise the dream or not, doesn't matter. It's the striving that keeps us alive, feeling energised and making a positive difference to the world. Tell me something that would ignite a flicker of interest or excitement in you—anything at all, and we'll make it happen."

"I just can't think of anything," he said.

"I've been going out of my mind trying to find things you might be interested in. But it's not up to me to hand you something on a platter."

Dad remained silent.

"Isn't there one small thing you'd like to do? Go to the Blue Mountains? Volunteer to do charity work? Go to a concert or a movie? I have no idea. You have to tell me." I crossed my fingers that it wouldn't involve Marko.

He thought for a long time. Then a faint trace of animation registered across his face but quickly faded.

"It would be nice to see my cousin in Belgrade one last time before I died," he ventured, almost apologetically. "I haven't seen her in 30 years."

"You'd like to visit cousin Milica in Belgrade?" I echoed.

He hesitated. "Yes, I think I would … but … how?"

"We'll get on a plane and in 24 hours we're there," I replied. Dad looked at me incredulously.

"Would you really want to go?" he asked.

"Absolutely!"

Belgrade was not at the top of my list of must-revisit cities, but if it was something my father wanted, we were going. *I* was excited about the prospect of Dad being excited. Excitement was synonymous with motivation. If he was excited about seeing cousin Milica, it would switch on his brain and motivate him to do things related to the trip. And his new-found enthusiasm would spill into other areas of life.

Aspirations turn on our brain cells much more powerfully than needs—*wanting* to do something activates more of our brain cells than *needing* to do something. Until now, my father had only been doing things because I'd told him he needed to do them. In addition, Dad would receive a long-overdue dose of dopamine and acetylcholine in his brain, two of the neurotransmitters secreted when we experience pleasure or excitement and which enhance our alertness and capacity for learning.

I began searching the Internet for flights. The fares were outrageous, but with my father on board, we were unstoppable—despite the best efforts of the passport office, travel insurance company and airlines to stop us.

Passport

For fast-acting relief, try slowing down.
Lily Tomlin

My mother loved travelling, especially to New York, Las Vegas, San Francisco, Hawaii and New Orleans. She was captivated by bright lights, tall buildings, colourful costumes and cabarets. It goes without saying that Fifth Avenue in Manhattan was her idea of paradise. Dad tagged dutifully along.

"Can you give me your passport, please?" I asked my father, as I began a checklist for our trip.

"I don't know where it is," he replied.

"Where do you keep all your important documents?"

"I don't know. Your mother looked after all that."

"Might it be in her bedside drawer?"

"Maybe."

Maybe not. We turned the entire house inside out and found no trace of a passport. I felt mild panic. We were flying to Belgrade in less than a month and the length of my to-do list was inversely proportional to the length of my fuse.

"Maybe my passport has expired," Dad suggested.

"I know for a fact that you renewed your passport two years ago," I snapped. "We'll have to apply for a new one. As if I haven't got enough to do."

Down at the post office, Brett reviewed the application form.

"Not so fast," he warned. "In the case of a lost passport, there needs to be a worldwide investigation to make sure that no-one is using it under false pretences. Identity theft is a threat to our security, both here and overseas."

"My father's passport isn't lost," I explained. "It's somewhere in the house but we just can't find it."

"If you can't find it, how can you be sure it's in the house? It might have been stolen," Brett persisted.

"My mother kept all important documents in a very safe place, but she's not around for us to ask where that is," I clarified. "We end up finding everything about a month after we need it."

"I'm sorry, but there's no avoiding the additional lost passport fee on top of the normal application fee. You'll also have to wait four weeks for the old passport to be cleared of fraudulent use. Then we can process the new application."

"But we don't have four weeks! We fly out in 23 days!"

"Four weeks is the worst-case scenario. Twenty-three days should be fine."

I felt sick. Walking out of the post office, I had a flashback to four years ago when I was planning a trip to Vietnam from Brisbane. Spookily, it was also 23 days before leaving when things started getting hairy.

Everything for Vietnam had been organised but it suddenly occurred to me that I hadn't asked about visa requirements. I presumed my travel agent would have said something if I needed one, but just to be sure, I rang her.

"Of course you need a visa for Vietnam," she stated. "Haven't you organised one?"

"No, I thought that was *your* job," I impugned.

"Well, we'd better get onto it straightaway. You need to allow three weeks because there's no Vietnamese Consulate in Brisbane, so your passport and application form have to go to Sydney."

"But I'm flying out in three weeks."

"You'd better come in and see me before five this afternoon."

I raced home from work, collected my passport, had obligatory mug shots taken and got to the travel agent before 5 pm. I thrived on fast living. While I was filling out the visa form, I saw in bold print that I needed six months' validity on my passport, which expired in just over six months. I mentioned my luck to the travel agent.

"Your passport has to be valid for six months from the time you enter the country," she confirmed.

"I arrive on 28 July, leaving five months and three weeks' validity on my passport. That should be near enough, shouldn't it?"

"No, it needs to be a full six months or you won't be issued a visa."

"Are you sure?" I didn't believe her. "Can you ring someone and find out?"

She rang someone and found out. I needed at least six months' validity on my passport; five months and three weeks wouldn't cut it.

"Don't tell me I need to get a new passport before I can apply for a visa?" I pleaded.

"I'm afraid so." Her composure was beginning to grate on me.

"Would you mind downloading a passport application form for me?"

On the Australian Passport website, we were greeted by a short, friendly note: *Due to technical difficulties, it is not possible to download passport application forms at this time. We apologise for any inconvenience.*

"So where am I going to get a form?"

"At the post office."

It was now 5.20 pm. There was a post office in Brisbane CBD that stayed open until 5.30 pm. Breaking all conceivable traffic laws and parking rules, I reached the post office at 5.31 pm. I could see customers inside but the doors were locked. I slipped inside when a customer left, but a staff member was soon escorting me out. I explained my situation but to no avail. While I was deep breathing, I remembered there was a post office in West End that closed at 6 pm. Why hadn't I thought of that in the first place? More Bangkok-style driving and I found myself at West End post office at 5.55 pm. I blurted out my request to the woman behind the counter.

"I'm sorry, passport renewal forms are not available at post offices. We only have *new* passport application forms. For renewals you have to contact the Passport Office and have it sent out to you. Allow 72 hours to receive the form. Here's the phone number."

I suddenly had empathy for vandals. I rang the number, explained my predicament and was given an appointment at the passport office the following afternoon, where I'd receive a renewal form in exchange for my old passport and appropriate photos. Luckily, I could use the same photos I'd had taken earlier that day for my visa.

I arrived for my appointment at 3.15 pm and handed over my old passport and my new photos.

"I'm sorry, these photos are unacceptable. Your face is one millimetre too small."

"You're kidding, aren't you?" I wasn't in the mood for humour.

"No, I'm not kidding. See this piece of clear plastic I'm holding over your photo? Your chin and forehead have to sit between these two black lines." I couldn't argue with the fact that my chin was one millimetre too high.

"Does it really matter?" Yesterday, a matter of one week had sealed my fate; today it was one millimetre.

"Yes, it does matter. You'll have to go and get the photos done again. I'll see when I can get you another appointment. How about Tuesday next week?" he offered.

"How about in 15 minutes?" I entreated. The photo place was a five-minute sprint away.

"We close at 4 pm. If you can get back before then I'll try and fit you in."

Knocking several cappuccinos into unsuspecting laps along the way, I made it to the photo shop and very politely informed them they'd be taking my photo again, free of charge, since the original was not acceptable to the passport office.

"But yesterday you said the photo was for a visa, not a passport," the photographer objected. "You don't have to be as precise with a visa photo. If you'd said you wanted a passport photo I'd have made your face the correct size."

After some quick bargaining, we agreed that I'd pay half the usual price for passport photos and I made it back to the passport office by 3.54 pm. I proudly presented the photos and renewal form to the man at the counter.

"What are all these brown marks smudged across the page?" he asked.

"I don't know," I lied. A cut on my finger had started to bleed while I was filling out the form. I'd left a trail of smudged blood all the way down the page.

"Sorry, this form is unacceptable. You'll have to fill out another one. And we close in one minute."

Wrapping a wad of toilet paper around my hand, I did it in 30 seconds.

"Your passport will be ready in three weeks."

"I need it in three days."

"Then you can pay the priority processing fee of $75. This guarantees a turnaround time of 48 hours."

I was already paying the priority processing fee for the visa, so why not for the passport as well? Two days later, I picked up my new passport and ran all the way to the travel agent. I handed her the relevant paperwork and a cheque for $72. She'd warned me that payment could only be made by cash or cheque.

"Personal cheques are not acceptable," she shook her head.

"Tell me this is a bad joke."

It was now after 5 pm. The travel agent agreed to wait while I ran to the nearest ATM. As I sprinted past a newsagent, I remembered that it was my mother's birthday the following day.

With all the excitement of the last week, I'd forgotten to send her a card. I briefly contemplated the relative repercussions of being late for the travel agent versus being late for my mother's birthday. I went inside and bought a card.

After writing some loving words at the counter, I stuck a stamp on the envelope and ran to a post box, half a block away. I hastily pulled open the lid and threw in the card—why I didn't just push the card through the slot, I have no idea. As the lid was closing, it caught on my black coral bangle (a gift from my mother), pulled it off my hand and dragged it into the post box. I heard a clunk as it fell inside. I stared at the mailbox in disbelief—but had to get back to the travel agent.

Once the passport saga was over, I rang Australia Post to explain what had happened to my bangle. I suggested the simplest way to get it back was to meet the postman when he came to collect the mail.

"Absolutely not!" was the adamant reply. "It's illegal to tamper with mail."

"I'm not tampering with mail; I'm merely retrieving my property."

"Once anything goes into a post box, it becomes mail."

"But it's not in an envelope and there's no stamp on it."

"That's irrelevant. Ring the Dead Letter Office tomorrow and ask them to look for it among the other incorrectly addressed mail."

There was no arguing, and despite numerous phone calls to the Dead Letter Office, the bangle was never found. I'm still on the lookout for a woman related to a postman wearing a black coral bangle.

Unravelling

The greatest weapon against stress is our ability to choose one thought over another.
William James

Reminiscing about passport dilemmas only compounded my frustrations in the present. It's amazing how things we dwell on seem to magnify. I'm not exactly sure what set me on a downhill slide. It was as though I woke up one morning seeing the world through the lens of "too hard". Things started becoming a drain and a strain. Tasks that should have taken half an hour ended up taking half a day. I was being drawn into a vortex of negativity, fuelled by my newly acquired mantra of "This is not fair!" Situations I would previously have labelled as "interesting challenges", I now viewed as "major headaches". Minor inconveniences became annoying problems. Opportunities for learning became stressful setbacks. Curiosity disintegrated into cantankerousness.

One afternoon, Dad came home from Marko's house reeking of cigarette smoke.

"You've been smoking!" I accused.

"I only had one puff," my father responded defensively.

"I don't believe you! Don't you dare start smoking again!" I was furious. My father had been a heavy smoker a decade ago, until combined pressure from his cardiologist, GP and my mother finally wore him down.

"Calm down. One cigarette now and again isn't going to make any difference."

"You wanna make a bet? If I catch you smoking again, I'm getting on the next plane to Brisbane and I'm not coming back! That's how much difference it's going to make! Every cigarette increases your risk of having a stroke, and smokers are 70 per cent more likely to develop dementia than non-smokers. I can't believe you'd have so little respect for me that you'd do something that goes against everything I'm trying to achieve for you!"

In retrospect, this was the problem: me trying to achieve things for my father, being too directive and not seeking enough of his input.

A few days later, I was sitting in the Qantas Club lounge, waiting for my return flight to Sydney from Adelaide. I was trying to fight off my exhaustion-induced grumpiness and growing resentment at having to prepare dinner for Dad as soon as I arrived home. My eyes came to rest on the smorgasbord laid out in the lounge. Robotically, I stood up, walked towards the food and piled several plates with pasta, potato salad, vegetable couscous and olives. I went back for rocket, sun-dried tomatoes, a few slices of rye bread and ham. I looked at the spread I'd collected and stealthily pulled out the empty plastic containers from lunch that I hadn't yet disposed of. Looking around to check that no-one was watching, I furtively filled them to the brim with my father's dinner. I smiled sweetly when a staff member came to clear away my six empty plates.

However, onboard the plane I broke into a cold sweat. What if there were security cameras in the lounge and I'd been caught pilfering food? What would I say if I was interrogated? Should I confess my crime before I was apprehended, so that I could plead for a lighter sentence? But who would I confess to? And who would look after my father if I were thrown in jail? I slipped in and out of fitful sleep until I was jolted awake by the thud of wheels on tarmac. I decided I was too tired to deal with my misdemeanours that evening and headed straight for home. I have not been contacted by Qantas and if anyone from the airline is reading this, please accept my profuse apologies and Dad's sincere compliments on your victuals.

For the rest of the week, I paid my karmic debt for the Qantas crime. The day I'd been in Adelaide, Dad crashed the car, so we were without a vehicle for seven days. Australia Post mistakenly stopped redirecting my mail from Brisbane to Sydney, so I was receiving daily hate-calls from irate people who thought I was ignoring their correspondence. All of my father's credit cards were cancelled because my mother was the primary card-holder, and he had no access to money other than via a bank teller—an hour-long excursion in the absence of a car. Dad's left hearing aid started playing up, which made it even harder for him to focus than usual. And I inadvertently cooked his mobile phone because I didn't see him leave it on the hot stove. I discovered the molten, misshapen mess when it was well beyond salvage, which added another thing to my to-do list. Although Dad rarely used the phone, he felt panicky without it and wanted a replacement as soon as possible.

The only thing stopping me from acts of vandalism was lack of time.

Meltdown

There cannot be a stressful crisis next week.
My schedule is already full.
Henry Kissinger

"Don't ever travel with someone who is over 75 years old and has a pre-existing heart condition unless you want to give *yourself* a pre-existing heart condition." I was SMSing banal advice to my friend, Sarah, while Dad and I sat in his cardiologist's waiting room. Three weeks ago we'd been at the same place for a routine check-up and all had been well. The cardiologist had even reduced my father's medications—which was precisely the reason the insurance company refused to accept his cardiology assessment of three weeks ago. They wanted a cardiology report on whether or not Dad's condition had remained stable after the dosage change. The fact that I was with my father every day, was myself a doctor and could verify that his health hadn't changed didn't satisfy the insurer. The cardiologist had to write an updated report confirming that Dad was as fit to travel now as he had been three weeks ago. Only then would they allow me to purchase travel insurance at extortionate rates. If we weren't going to Los Angeles to visit Dean, Mum's childhood friend, on our way to Serbia, I wouldn't have bothered. However, if Dad ended up in hospital in the United States, we'd need to mortgage the house to afford it.

While I was pocketing a hastily penned report from an unimpressed cardiologist, I received a reply from Sarah: "I think you need to attend The Happiness Conference at Darling Harbour with me next week. You'll learn how to tap into your own constant, inner source of joy and peace, regardless of your external circumstances."

"No time," I responded.

"Make time," she insisted.

"I'm so busy, I'm looking to outsource brushing my teeth."

Sarah offered to bring two days' worth of food for my father (complete with assembly and heating instructions), so that I'd be able to attend the conference. She topped my gratitude list that week.

Only half an hour into the conference, I was already feeling happier. The event was run by Vajrayana Tibetan Buddhist Institute, which is dedicated to providing practical solutions to the problems and suffering of daily life. Sarah was right: this was exactly what I needed.

The first speaker was Professor Barbara Fredrickson, an American psychologist and pioneering researcher of positive emotions. Professor Fredrickson explained how positive emotions not only feel good, they change the architecture and functioning of our brains. When we experience positive emotions—such as joy, love, contentment, gratitude, compassion, forgiveness, enthusiasm, calm and connectedness—we take in more information from our environment and we're better able to view things in context. Positivity raises our ability to see the bigger picture, to remember details, to generate options and to bounce back from setbacks.

Professor Fredrickson was about to tell us how we could increase our positivity, when my mobile phone started vibrating. I was surprised to see my home number on the screen—Dad should have been at Men's Shed by now. Steve had agreed to pick him up, despite it being out of his way. What could have gone wrong? I'd written all the instructions on the whiteboard; Dad's yellow lunchbox was clearly labelled and sitting on the usual shelf in the fridge; plastic cutlery was sticky-taped to the container; and a yellow serviette was next to his bag. Something must have happened to Steve.

"What's wrong?" I whispered, so as not to disturb the people around me.

"Nothing's wrong," answered my father. "Do you know where my black address book is?"

"No, I don't. Why aren't you at Men's Shed? Didn't Steve turn up?"

"Yes, Steve turned up but I told him I didn't feel like going today."

"You *what*? Are you saying you sent Steve away?"

"Yes."

"How *could* you? Do you have any idea how much effort it takes to organise someone to give you a lift? Do you know how inconvenient it was for Steve to come this morning? Do you think everyone in this world is just sitting around at your beck and call?"

I was shouting. The speaker looked in my direction as she continued her useless drivel—something about "becoming the observer of our emotions ... Despite crashing waves and raging storms on the surface of the sea, the depths of the ocean remain calm and still." A minute ago, this speaker had been my hero; now I was dismissing everything she said. We don't see things as they are—we see things as *we* are. I cringe as I recall the events of that morning.

"I've had it with you!" I unloaded. "I bust my gut from morning till night being your servant, your housekeeper, your chef, your chauffeur, your doctor, your nurse, your diversional therapist, your social secretary, your personal trainer and your life coach, while *you* won't get off your skinny backside to do a single thing unless I put a hand grenade under it! I had no idea it was possible to be so devoid of initiative! You never notice a thing that needs doing. When we arrive home from a trip you just plonk yourself on the couch and turn on the TV. How do you think your suitcase gets unpacked? Fairies? And do you think I enjoy playing treasure hunt for your socks and undies whenever I do a load of washing? Why do things have to be strewn from one end of the house to the other?"

I took a breath and Dad countered patiently, "I try my best to help you. Instead of going to Men's Shed, I fixed the hinge on the bathroom cupboard and now I just want some time out." I was only vaguely aware of Sarah steering me out of the auditorium as I continued my tirade.

"Your whole life has been time out! The bathroom cupboard was a five-minute, optional job for you to do *after* Men's Shed. Why do you think I organise things for you? It isn't for *my* benefit. My life would be a lot easier if I left you to do nothing all day every day. You keep asking me to help you improve your memory but you object to every single thing I propose. I'm doing everything in my power to boost your brain, to get you fit and to give you purpose, but you don't make a shred of effort in return!"

I don't know how long I ranted. Dad said nothing more. When I awoke from the spell, I found myself in a disabled persons toilet. Later I discovered that Sarah had led me there because it was the only place I couldn't be heard from the auditorium.

I was angry.

I was angry with my father for his apathy, his inertia and his lack of motivation. I was angry at his incapacity to look after himself and for his expectation that I'd take care of everything. I was angry with my father for not wanting to make new friends.

I was angry at his defeatist attitude. I was angry at his negative self-talk and his uncritical acceptance of ageism. I was angry with my *mother* for allowing him to stay home and do nothing, while *she* led an active professional, social and charitable life. I was angry that I'd wasted years of my life being angry with my mother. I was angry that I'd never sat down and asked my mother her stories, her passions, her motivations and her dreams. I was angry that I learnt things about my mother after she died that I should have known while she was alive. I was angry with *myself* for not having "worked out" my father by now and for not having the skills to motivate him. I was angry with myself for not embracing this opportunity for "selfless service". I was angry with myself for not being able to let everything "wash over me".

I was angry with myself for being angry.

I became conscious of the anger as a pile of bricks compressing my chest, a physical weight pinning me down, oppressing me, crushing me, paralysing me. The sensation was so intense, I could barely breathe. I used all my strength to force air into my lungs. The exertion detonated my lacrimal glands and I burst into tears. By the time I returned to the auditorium, it was almost lunchtime.

"Are you OK?" asked Sarah gently.

"I have a sore throat," I croaked. "I just don't know what to do any more."

"Maybe you don't need to do any more," she speculated.

"I don't understand."

"Maybe it's time you stopped *doing* and just started listening." Sarah's tone remained compassionate. "You're allowed to not have all the answers. You have permission to press Pause and to wait for life to show you the next step. You might be an authority on the brain, but you aren't an authority on the totality of human experience, on grief, on loss, on self-determination or on anyone else's internal world. You're used to dealing with individuals and groups who *want* to improve their health and their quality of life. Your patients and clients see purpose and value in making an effort to change their behaviour, but your father is in a completely different place. Three months ago he went through the most devastating experience of his life. He lost his partner of 43 years, along with his purpose, his role and his identity. He no longer sees where he fits into the scheme of things. Life, as he knew it, evaporated. He must have been terrified in every fibre of his being, not to mention the inconceivable pain he'd still be suffering. He feels totally betrayed by life. It was never in his game plan that his wife would die before he did. It was never in his game plan that he wouldn't have grandchildren. It was never in his game plan to become dependent on his daughter. And in the midst of all this unfairness, you bounce in wearing tights and tank tops, expecting him to pump weights at the gym! Can you see how it might seem absurd and pointless to him?

"It's like a mother pushing her child to do music lessons," Sarah continued. "Yes, learning a musical instrument is a great thing to do on many levels. But some kids are simply not inclined to play music. You have to let them follow their own passions and interests, or everyone ends up being miserable and resenting each other."

"But *my* 'child' isn't interested in anything!"

"All you can do is offer your dad a smorgasbord of activities and let him decide what, if anything, arouses his interest. Force, manipulation, bribery and constant negotiation won't work. It'll wear you out and you won't achieve anything in the long run.

There are infinite possibilities for a fulfilling life. I know *you* value health and high-energy living, but that's not the path for everyone.

"The attitude we bring to everything we do is more important than the actual doing. The means don't justify the ends because the means *are* the end in any given moment. You keep saying that if someone hates exercise and anticipates it with dread, they elevate their cortisol levels and undo the good they're trying to achieve. If your father doesn't like going to Men's Shed, don't force him to go. Isn't one of your mantras 'fun not force'? Having said that, I think your dad *did* need a push at the start. He needed someone to help him re-engage with life. But he's no longer suicidal and he comes across as switched-on and animated. If you allow him things that give him pleasure—TV, pavlova and pottering around the house doing what you consider to be 'nothing'—you might find that he becomes motivated to do a little more. The more you push, the more he'll resist. If you over-function, he'll under-function. You can't know what's going on inside his head. He may be processing his grief, appreciating the present moment or living in a fantasy world. It doesn't matter. Whatever it is, it's what *he* needs. He's doing the best he can with the resources and the understanding he has. Isn't that what we're all doing? Aren't we all just doing the best we can, given the life experiences we've had?"

What did I do to deserve a friend like Sarah? She hadn't finished yet.

"You can't barge into your father's life expecting him to take on your values. I know you have a barrage of scientific data supporting your world view, but that's only one aspect of human existence. Love, kindness, compassion and unconditional acceptance are more healing than diet, exercise or any structured activity you devise.

"Just try *being* there for him. Not judging him, not questioning him and not trying to figure him out. *Be* there for him, for no other reason than to *be* there. Don't be looking for ways to motivate him to live what you consider a fulfilling and meaningful life. That's not your call; that's his call. By all means offer him health information, but trust him to intuitively know what's best for him. There's no pre-determined best way to live. We figure it out as we go, each one of us. Beyond preserving his life and showing him respect as an equal, you have no right to determine how he should live. You don't know what's best for him as an evolving human being. Trust the life force within him to guide him—and to show you, when you stop to listen, how you can best support him. Your role is to support him, not subjugate him.

"Give him the gift your mother never gave: self-determination. Trusting him to make decisions for himself will feed his spirit and his self-confidence enormously. What caused the most friction between you and your mother?"

"She always thought she knew what was best for me and for Dad," I replied. "And she'd force it on us, whether we wanted it or not, all in the name of love." I shook my head. "How could I be such a hypocrite? How could I have had such a huge blind spot?"

"It's hard to have perspective when you're caught in the middle of something," Sarah smiled. "In my experience, we can never judge the actions of others because we never know their whole story. The very thing we perceive as weakness might actually be an expression of strength, a survival instinct. You'll do your head in trying to 'figure out' your dad, or anyone else for that matter.

"Just accept him."

Part VI
Love Comes Above

The only way to understand someone is to love them.
And then it isn't necessary to understand them.

Unknown

Responsibility

*We are all faced with a series of great opportunities brilliantly
disguised as impossible situations.*
Charles R. Swindoll

Acceptance is easier said than done.

About four months after my mother died, she came to Marko
in a dream. She told Marko to reassure my father that he had
nothing to worry about, that he would always have someone to
take care of him, and that he'd live past 90 years old. Dad was
surprised that my mother would go to Marko, rather than relay
the message directly to him. I was surprised that my mother
hadn't told Marko to buzz off.

A week later, Marko's car started leaking oil and he needed $600
from my father to get it fixed. This prompted a serious discussion
between me and Dad about money and friends.

"I think it's lovely that you're able to help Marko out," I began,
trying not to hiss, "but what concerns me is a friendship that
becomes contaminated by money."

"Marko and his wife are struggling to make ends meet on their
pension," my father explained. "I don't need much money and
you're a doctor, so we can afford to help out the less fortunate."

"Yes, we can. That's why I sponsor a child in Cambodia and
regularly donate to several charities. But giving money to friends
is different. It calls into question the nature of the friendship."

"If Marko doesn't have a car to drive, how will they go shopping
and do what they need to do?" Dad demanded.

"There's public transport," I offered. "And don't they have children? Maybe one of them could help out once in a while?"

"His children have their own children to look after. Don't be so mean-spirited," he chided.

"Really? So if I had my own children, you wouldn't expect me to come and help you? I'm not being mean-spirited; I just don't want you to be taken advantage of."

Dad was immovable on the subject. It struck me as a curious coincidence that we were leaving for overseas in less than a fortnight and $600 would average out to, let's see, roughly $75 a week for Marko while we were away… I made two appointments for the first business day after our return from overseas: one with my parents' solicitor and one with my parents' bank manager.

All the talk of money reminded me to follow up on the holiday and sick pay owed to my mother. Dad kept urging me to take care of it, so I rang her former workplace to find out what to do.

"There's a cheque written out to the Estate of the Deceased, waiting to be picked up," said Justine from the accounts office.

"Would you be able to post it to us, please?"

"No, I'm afraid not. As the sole beneficiary, your father has to pick up the cheque in person or write a letter authorising you to pick it up for him. You'd need to bring a certified copy of his photo ID."

"Why so much fuss?"

"You don't want a cheque for $29 978 getting lost in the mail, do you?"

"Oh. Of course not. It won't be a problem." I hadn't realised it would be such a large amount. I organised the paperwork and had the cheque in hand that Friday afternoon. I went straight to the bank and deposited the cheque into Dad's account.

"You didn't lose it on the way, did you?" my father joked that evening.

"It's all good," I said. "We can check your account balance on the Internet when the cheque clears in three days' time." We did. There was no record of the cheque.

"We'll look again tomorrow. Sometimes it takes a day longer," I reassured him.

"Why don't you ring the bank to make sure?"

"Because I'm sure," I replied impatiently. "Just wait another 24 hours." We did. There was still no record of the transaction.

"Ring the bank," Dad pleaded. I rang the bank.

"Sorry, there's no record of $29 978 being deposited into that account," Nancy, the bank clerk, announced.

"Well, there must be because I'm holding the deposit receipt in my hand." I spoke through clenched teeth.

"I'm very sorry. I have nothing in my records," she repeated.

I began to feel sick, a horrid, empty, nauseating, churning-pit-in-the-stomach kind of feeling, at an intensity I had never before experienced.

"OK, let's go through everything again slowly," I began. Then I noticed something that saw the churning reach new levels. The account number on the deposit slip didn't match Dad's account number. I looked from one number to the other and back again. There was no resemblance between the two numbers. Why hadn't I noticed this on the day?

"Well, there's the problem!" Nancy chirped. "You deposited the cheque into another account."

"But that other account doesn't belong to my father—or to anyone else I know," I exclaimed. "And I distinctly recall handing the correct account number to the teller in writing. I also still happen to have *that* piece of paper. So how did the money end up in someone else's account?"

"I don't know."

"Well, I suggest you find out and transfer it back into my father's account."

"I'm afraid I can't do that," Nancy apologised. "I can't just take money out of someone else's account and put it into *your* account. Besides, I don't know who the other account belongs to."

"Then go and ask the teller who *mis*handled the transaction whose account it is!" I was starting to lose my composure.

"Certainly, I'll do that," said Nancy. "But could you also ring the people who issued the cheque and get back to me with the cheque details, please? That will make it easier for me to track it down."

"OK," I replied tersely. "You do *your* bit and I'll do *my* bit, and I expect a call from you within 30 minutes." I hung up.

With trepidation I rang Justine from the accounts office. She was away from her desk, so I left a message to return my call as soon as possible. In the meantime, I had to take Dad to his appointment with the audiologist. I kept looking at my mobile phone, anticipating calls from Nancy and Justine. No-one rang until we were in the car on our way home. The lights had just turned green and the traffic was starting to move. I glanced down briefly to reach for my phone, simultaneously inserting the earpiece, but when I looked up, the car in front had stopped. I hit the brakes but it was too late.

We tapped the numberplate of the car in front and came to a jerky standstill. The driver jumped out of the car, looked at his numberplate and began swearing. I approached him ruefully. There wasn't a scratch on my father's car and barely a dent in his. The other driver launched into a verbal tirade, way out of proportion with the damage. He moved away to "ring the police" (maybe he just pretended to do this, in order to intimidate me), but I couldn't hear what he was saying. Then we coldly exchanged details and he assured me I'd be hearing from his insurance company.

"I'm really sorry," I said to Dad as I got back in the car. I was shaky and tearful—not because of my carelessness or the extra hassles I'd created for myself, but because of the menacing nature of the other driver. There was no need for his vitriol.

"It's no big deal," Dad said comfortingly. "Accidents happen." He paused for a moment. "At that talk in Brisbane, you said that multi-tasking doubles the likelihood of making a mistake, and that just reaching for something in the car increases your risk of having a car accident by nine times. You can now tell people that you've personally put this to the test and proved it to be true."

"Thanks," I said, smiling through my tears.

As soon as we arrived home, my phone rang again. It was Justine, and I apologetically explained what had happened at the bank.

"Is it too late for you to cancel the cheque and re-issue another one?" I asked.

"Wait a moment and let me see what's happened at our end." I appreciated her composure and patience. "Well, well!" she exclaimed. "What's the account number you say the money was deposited into?" I gave it to her. "That's *our* account number! Your bank deposited the money back into our account instead of putting it in yours!" We both burst out laughing.

"The bank will pay for this," I declared. "Along with compensation for the anxiety and emotional distress I've suffered as a result. Not to mention the car accident I had because I was trying to answer the phone when the bank was ringing me!"

"Good luck!" Justine said. "And thanks for the great dinner party story." We'd become best mates.

I took great delight informing Nancy of the bank's incompetence, and she apologised profusely. She promised to take everything in hand and resolve the issue as quickly as possible. I suggested they sack the bank teller; Nancy said the teller's supervisor would be informed and appropriate action would be taken.

When I hung up, Dad looked at me reprovingly. "That wasn't very generous of you, asking for the teller to be sacked."

"Do you have any idea how much angst she caused me?"

"You hypocrite!" my father accused. "You preach that our response to something is always our choice. No-one can *make* you feel anything. If you get angry about something, that's your choice. If you let something wash over you and not waste your energy getting worked up about it, that's also your choice. You're *choosing* to make a big deal out of a woman at the bank making a rectifiable mistake. It isn't as though she did it on purpose. Maybe she was having a bad day. Maybe she'd just found out that her boyfriend was cheating on her. Maybe her young child had kept her up all night and she was tired. Everyone is doing the best they can—just like you were doing your best when you hit that car today. The accident could have been avoided if you hadn't reached for the phone. But I understand you were anxious about this whole cheque fiasco. That's why I told you it was OK. You had your reasons; the bank teller probably had hers. And the driver who went off his head might also have had his reasons. Since everyone has their reasons, everyone has to take responsibility for their actions. Otherwise how far back in history do you want to point the finger of blame?"

"I was ..."

"Tomorrow I'd like you to go to the bank and take Nancy a present. Thank her for resolving the situation so quickly. Then go to the bank teller who made the mistake and give her a present. Tell her you understand how badly she must be feeling and that you'll make sure she doesn't get sacked."

"But ..." I began to protest.

"Trust me: if you do that, neither of them will ever forget the incident, especially the bank teller. It's just possible that it will turn her into the best, most reliable teller the bank has. She'll be the person *least* likely to ever make a mistake like that again. Best of all is how *you'll* feel. Tell me all about it when you come home."

I wanted to hug my father. I did exactly as he asked and felt genuine goodwill towards both women at the bank. I felt a real lightness driving home.

"You see," Dad beamed. "Life isn't about 'being right' all the time. Isn't it more important to be happy?"

Chick Magnet

The final week before leaving for overseas was nothing short of an obstacle race.

Two months' worth of medications had to be procured. "Make sure you leave all the tablets in their original, sealed boxes," advised the pharmacist, "otherwise Customs might think what you're carrying is illegal."

An hour after we arrived home, Dad declared, "I've had a great idea. I've opened all my medications and put them into a single, small container, so we don't have to carry so many boxes."

We spent the next hour fishing all the boxes out of the recycling bin and replacing the medications. Now they definitely looked tampered with. I crossed my fingers that the letter from Dad's GP, listing all his medications, would see us through.

We also had to buy presents for all our relatives and friends in Serbia and Los Angeles. "I have a great idea!" exclaimed Dad. I braced myself. "Let's get everyone in Belgrade an electric blanket," he continued. "I'll bet they don't have electric blankets over there, and the winters are bitterly cold." He was clearly very pleased with his proposal.

"Electric blankets are a very thoughtful suggestion," I began. "My only concern is that they'll take up too much room in our luggage."

"We're going in summer, so we don't need to pack many clothes. I'm sure we can make them fit." For once I hoped the dementia would kick in and he'd forget about the electric blankets by the time we went shopping.

We also both rewrote our wills, in the event that neither of us returned from the trip—if I wasn't around, who would my father leave the house and Tupperware to? What concerned me most was that I wouldn't be around to contest Marko's share.

In the middle of all the travel preparations, an irresistible opportunity arose. A friend of a friend owned a dog, which had just given birth to 12 puppies, all needing loving homes. The puppies would be weaned in two to three months, ready for collection precisely when we returned from overseas. It was meant to be.

Pets have long been observed to improve physical, mental and emotional wellbeing. A puppy would help to give Dad a sense of purpose and responsibility. A puppy would give him comfort and companionship (and maybe competition for Marko). A puppy would meet my father's need to be needed because he'd have to feed and walk it every day. Walking the dog would be an added incentive to keep fit and an opportunity for socialising with other dog owners. A puppy would induce neighbourhood children to visit, and Dad would either have to supervise them or entertain their parents.

A puppy would deliver Dad joy and affection and be better at unconditional love and acceptance than I was. And a puppy was a surefire chick magnet.

Packing: Take 3

We cannot hold a torch to light another's path without
brightening our own.
Ben Sweetland

Maybe—just maybe—following typed instructions was not my father's preferred modus operandi. I was determined that packing for Serbia would not see our house transformed into a street stall; on the contrary, it would be an opportunity to **Turn Stress into Success**. Thankfully, the electric blankets had not been mentioned again; the relatives would receive jewellery and scarves.

"This is the moment you've been waiting for!" I announced on the eve of our departure. Dad looked mystified. "It's time to pack!"

"Show me the itinerary," my father requested for the twentieth time that week.

"Tomorrow we catch a plane to Los Angeles. Dean will be waiting for us at the airport when we arrive. We stay with him and his wife for three weeks before flying to Belgrade via Munich. When we arrive in Belgrade, Cousin Milica and entourage will meet us. We stay with them for five weeks and then fly straight home to Sydney. Now, let's decide what you'd like to take."

Together we selected underwear, socks, clothes and shoes for all occasions. Together we chose books for him to read in planes and airports. Together we placed things neatly in his suitcase. Together we put irreplaceable things in his hand luggage. "Together" was a much easier, friendlier and more confidence-boosting way to do things. Duh! Why hadn't I thought of it before?

Bon Voyage

*Praise and blame, gain and loss, pleasure and sorrow come and
go like the wind. To be happy, rest like a giant tree
in the midst of them all.*
Buddha

We got off to a flying start at Sydney airport (pun intended).
After putting our hand luggage through security screening, Dad
asked me to wait so he could put his passport back into his bag.

"You don't *have* your passport," I said impatiently. "I'm carrying
both of them."

"Then what's this?" he blinked quizzically, waving a passport.

"You've picked up someone else's passport!" I shrieked. "Quick,
we have to give it back!" It wasn't hard to identify the distressed
young man having a panicked discussion with airport security. I
apologetically handed him the passport before diving for cover
among the crowds.

I took every conceivable precaution to prevent my father from
getting a deep vein thrombosis (DVT) while flying: loose clothing,
compression stockings, use of the footrest, no dehydrating fluids,
half-hourly foot flexion exercises, and second hourly walks up
and down the aisles. Wearing compression stockings, which are
tight around the ankles and gradually exert less pressure up the
leg, are the single most effective preventative measure against
DVT. Dad didn't like them.

I nagged the entire flight. "Try and sit so that your legs are as
stretched out as possible ... Try and slide your bottom forward,
so the angle between your legs and abdomen is more open ...
Sorry to wake you up every half hour, but these ankle rotations

could save your life … Stretch your neck and roll your shoulders; it improves your overall circulation … If you have any pain or swelling in either of your calves, tell me straight away … Or any shortness of breath or chest pain … "

"What has that got to do with a clot in my leg?"

"A piece of the clot in your leg vein can break off and lodge in a blood vessel in your lungs. It's called a pulmonary embolus and it can kill you." When we stepped off the plane, I noticed something white hanging out of my father's hand luggage. They were his compression stockings.

"I took them off to give my legs a rest," Dad explained.

"When?"

"A little while ago."

"On the plane? What exactly do you mean by 'a little while ago'?"

"Towards the end of the flight. But I'm fine and we're off the plane, so you don't have to worry."

"Yes, I do! You can get symptoms of a DVT up to a month after flying!" I stormed off to retrieve our checked luggage. "If you get a DVT I'll kill you."

"But you won't need to—didn't you say the clot would kill me?"

Respite

To be wronged is nothing, unless you continue to remember it.
Confucius

Dad did not develop a DVT after the flight—he developed a superficial vein thrombosis (SVT) instead.

An SVT is a blood clot in a superficial vein, rather than a deep one. It's usually accompanied by an inflammatory reaction (phlebitis), causing warmth and redness to the overlying skin. I noticed swelling and discolouration around my father's left ankle a few days after landing. The front of his lower leg was tender, and I could feel a firm, thickened, underlying vein. Unlike a DVT, an SVT is usually a benign, self-limiting condition, rarely throwing off emboli. However, sometimes an SVT can progress to adjacent deep veins and cause a DVT. Treatment is therefore aimed at relieving symptoms and preventing extension to deeper veins.

I added an anti-inflammatory drug to Dad's medications and gave him warm, soothing compresses. Long daily walks were mandatory to encourage good circulation, as was donning his compression stockings again.

"Since you didn't keep them on during the flight, you have to wear them now," I reproached.

"You're mean," he sulked.

"This is not punishment. The stockings improve blood flow and help to dissolve the clot." By the end of a week, everything had resolved and I heaved a massive sigh of relief.

The rest of our time in Los Angeles passed uneventfully. During the first few nights, my father intermittently woke up agitated and disoriented, but he settled back down quickly. One night he came to my room almost in tears. My mother had come to him in a dream (I guess she wasn't in the mood to visit Marko) and reprimanded him for taking me for granted. I don't believe in dead people coming back to reprimand their spouses but I said a quiet prayer of thanks to my mother nonetheless.

LA provided the respite I very much needed. Dean and his wife, Anna, catered for all Dad's needs, leaving me to write and go to the gym every day. I felt rejuvenated and ready to tackle whatever Serbia had to offer.

Freedom

Love life and life will love you back.
Love people and they will love you back.
Arthur Rubinstein

We managed to get through LA airport with marginally less drama than Sydney. As we were putting our things through security screening, Dad started taking off his hearing aids.

"You can leave them on," I instructed.

"No, I don't want them getting damaged," he fretted.

"They won't get damaged," I reassured him.

"No! They're very finely tuned and very expensive, and I don't want the X-rays interfering with them."

An official intervened to back me up. "Sir, it's no problem. We have people with hearing aids come through all the time and they always leave them on."

"No."

I took a deep breath. If we'd had the time and there hadn't been 34 impatient people in the queue behind us (I'd counted them while we were waiting), I'd have sat the official down and explained that people with compromised cognitive function sometimes get fixated on an idea, and there's no point reasoning with them unless you have a great deal of fortitude and an hour to spare. It's quicker and easier to go along with them and get the job done on their terms. As it was, Dad insisted the official examine his hearing aids manually without putting them through any sort of rays. In return for this favour, we had to undergo a comprehensive search for explosives, which involved opening every pocket of every bag and having a probe passed over every part of our luggage and person. That's when they noticed my father's half-full water bottle. I'd forgotten to empty it.

"Sorry, sir, you can't take this liquid through. You'll have to drink it or throw it out." Dad drank a third of the water and slipped the bottle back in his bag.

"No, you can't take *any* of it with you."

"The fact that I've just drunk some of it," my father reasoned, "and haven't dropped dead or exploded should indicate to you that it doesn't contain anything dangerous."

"I'm sorry, sir, those are the rules."

"But that's ridiculous. It's not logical. Oh, I get it—you think the explosive material is in the bottom half of the water and normal water was in the top half."

By now I'd done so much deep breathing I was surprised there was any oxygen left. I grabbed the water and drank the rest of it. If I ever have to go through LA airport again, I'll be wearing a disguise.

The 90-minute flight from Munich to Belgrade delivered the unexpected highlight of our trip thus far. I had closed my eyes to sleep when I suddenly felt a kiss on my cheek. I opened my eyes to see Dad smiling at me.

"Thanks," he said. Suddenly all the airport embarrassments faded into insignificance.

Try as we might, neither of us got any sleep during our 16 hours in the air, which meant we hadn't slept for more than 28 hours by the time we were mobbed at the airport by Dad's cousin, her two granddaughters and the boyfriend of one granddaughter.

I loved our hosts from the moment I met them. Dad's 83 year-old, graceful and remarkably wrinkle-free cousin was Milica. (I'd have to ask her how she kept her skin so smooth.) She had one child, a daughter called Gorica, who was currently with her husband in Moscow on business. Gorica had two daughters, Biljana and Nevena. Biljana, the eldest, had studied international law and was currently working in her father's business in Belgrade. She lived with her boyfriend, Milan, who worked at the same place and who was at the airport chaperoning the ladies. Her younger sister, Nevena, lived with grandmother Milica while studying architecture at Belgrade University.

In typical Serbian fashion, Dad and I were offered a four-course smorgasbord supper as soon as we arrived. I could barely keep my eyes open, but I managed to work my way through a stuffed cabbage roll (known as 'sarma'), a few teaspoons of yoghurt and 90 minutes of conversation before we were finally released to our quarters downstairs.

When I saw the sleeping arrangements, I was thrilled. Everything looked perfect. The self-contained area had three bedrooms, one each for me, my father and Nevena, and Dad and I had a bathroom, kitchenette and library of Cyrillic books to ourselves. What more could we possibly want?

Before collapsing into bed, I had to have a shower. That's when I noticed the unusual configuration of the bathroom. The door opened inwards, but only half way because it collided with the toilet. The advantage of this was that if I forgot to lock the door, no-one could just walk in and catch me doing my business—they'd slam the door into my knees before they could get in. As for the shower, it was perched at waist height against one wall, without surrounding walls or a shower curtain. Only a small dip in the floor with a white plastic stool underneath the tap told you that it was in fact the shower. OK, so I was meant to sit down and huddle under the showerhead or hold onto the detachable nozzle, making sure I aimed it away from the towels, toilet, mirror and lace curtains. In my hazy, somnolent state, I hoped I was up for the challenge. All went well until the very end when I dropped the nozzle and sprayed the entire bathroom floor with water, while chasing the snake-like, writhing tubing at my feet. When I turned off the taps, the nozzle jumped off its hook and knocked me forcefully on the head. I made a mental note to warn Dad of the potential hazards.

Furthermore, none of the rest of the downstairs doors closed properly. The door between the living area and Dad's bedroom jammed half way and wouldn't budge. The problem seemed to be an upward-sloping floor. Meanwhile, the door between our two bedrooms collided with my father's bed before it closed, so I was forced to wear industrial-strength ear plugs to block out his snoring.

But as I sank into bed, I was filled with peace and gratitude. All the minor inconveniences were a very small price to pay for a month of freedom from cooking, cleaning, washing, chauffeuring, grocery shopping, negotiating, personal training, paperwork and organising Dad's social life.

Internal Affairs

We are hard-wired for meaning. Where people are doing
something that has meaning, there is greater drive and energy.
Michael Rennie

Within 24 hours of arriving in Serbia, Dad and I had to present
to the Ministry for Internal Affairs with our passports and our
host, Milica, otherwise all three of us would be fined. The official
reason was "the safety and wellbeing of our visitors"; to me it
looked like a complete waste of time.

The Ministry was less than a kilometre from home, but on
account of Milica's severely arthritic hips and lack of a car, it
took us 40 minutes to walk there. It caused *me* pain watching her.
She took herself everywhere on foot, all the while maintaining an
attitude of pragmatic acceptance. How does one learn that kind
of acceptance?

We arrived to find five burly men in crisp, blue uniforms, crowded
into a tiny booth, which had an adjoining, equally minuscule
tearoom. One couple was already standing at the window.
During our 35-minute wait, I marvelled at the productivity of
each of the constabulary-like personnel. One man spent the entire
time making five cups of coffee—in fact, he hadn't finished by
the time we left. I have never seen anyone go to such laborious
lengths to make a cup of *instant* coffee. First he placed a heaped
teaspoon of Nescafé in a cup. Then he added a small amount
of boiling water and stirred and stirred and stirred until the
mixture formed a paste. Then he added a bit of sugar, stirred a
bit more, and then added a bit more sugar. Then he poured some
more water into the cup and stirred again. Finally, he topped it
up with milk and placed it in front of man #2, who had been
busily staring at a computer screen—not typing, not touching the

mouse, not even moving his eyes. He remained oblivious to the extraordinary beverage that had just been created for him.

The coffee maker then repeated the process with a second cup. This time he added a bit more sugar and did a bit more stirring than he had with the first cup, before placing it before man #3, who was serving the two people at the window. Actually, "serving" is a bit of a stretch. He was manually copying information from the woman's passport onto a small piece of cardboard. The speed of his writing was matched by the speed of the coffee-making. He too ignored the offering. Man #4 and man #5 leant against a wall sharing jokes. When man #4 received his coffee, he took one sip and said to the coffee maker, "This is cold. I can't drink it." Well, hello! I could have told him that. So the coffee maker switched on the kettle and started again. Maybe that's how he spent his entire day.

Finally, it was our turn to stand in front of the man with the unhurried pen. If it hadn't been for the entertainment his colleagues were providing, I would have ripped the pen out of his hand and filled out the card myself, especially since I had to watch him do it *three* times—once for me and twice for Dad. Twice in the second instance because when he got to the very last question, he made an error, deliberated over it for a few minutes, ripped up the card and started again. And Serbia wonders why they haven't been accepted into the EU. He finally handed us the credit-card sized documents and waved us away. I asked what we should do with them.

"Carry them with you at all times, along with your passports."

"Why?"

He looked at me as though I were a fool. "So that you can be identified."

"By whom?"

"By the police."

"Why would I have anything to do with the police?"

He was getting impatient. "In case anything happens."

"Such as?"

"I don't know. You need to go to a fortune-teller for that."

By now I was being dragged away by my father and Milica. Apparently everyone in Serbia has to carry ID cards in the event of something "untoward" happening.

"Such as?" I pursued.

"Such as a car accident or a coronary."

I managed to fend off my companions long enough to ask one more question. "Do you need to know when we leave the country?"

"Of course we do. Come back within 24 hours of your departure and we'll make a note of it."

"But I can give you that information now and save us another trip."

"I don't need to know now."

I was fervently bundled down the stairs. There was no way I would let Dad carry his passport with him. Nor was I going to accompany him everywhere he went with Milica. So I gave him a photocopy of his passport, folded the page, slotted the Serbian card between the folds and handed it to him. I watched as he placed it in his wallet.

"You'll carry that with you everywhere you go and always keep it safe," I charged him. I crossed my fingers very tightly.

Initiation

I shut my eyes in order to see.
Paul Gauguin

Whenever I arrive in a new town, I like to lace up my joggers and take in the local sights, and inner-city, suburban Belgrade offered plenty of sights. The houses had peeling grey or brown façades, with black stains and thick, rusting window bars. Most gardens featured broken cement, and the streets were pure rubble. More appropriate footwear would have been hiking boots.

The entire main drag was a construction site with not much construction happening. I surmised from the diligence of the workers that they were brothers of the staff at the Ministry for Internal Affairs. The footpath I was trying not to trip over, consisted of rocks, sand, gravel, steel and sharp, jutting edges, waiting to attack unwary pedestrians. No wonder everyone looked wary. Serbia was obviously not a mollycoddling or litigious nation. Back home, Workplace Health and Safety would have cordoned off the entire area and prohibited pedestrian access. Instead, people were hopping over slabs of cracked pavement, while ducking and weaving between cranes that dribbled dirt on their heads.

I wandered around fascinated until I stumbled (literally) upon a large park, complete with swimming pool, tennis courts, fitness centre, running oval, outdoor strength-training equipment and children's play zone. Excellent! I headed straight for the gym and asked to be shown the facilities. The chatty owner gave me a tour of the barbells, weight machines and jazzercise room, all the while with a cigarette dangling from the corner of his mouth. I asked about the cost of joining for a month: the equivalent of $30. No problem—tomorrow I'd bring the money and start training.

"Whoa! Not so fast. We don't re-open until September 15th," he informed me.

"Why not? I'll be back in Australia by then."

I received the first of many what-planet-are-you-from looks. "It's the summer holidays."

"So?"

"So we're on holidays."

"I see. Do you mean to tell me that every year you close over summer?"

"Of course."

Of course. I spent the next half-hour running around the oval and swinging from the outdoor chin-up bars.

The following evening I went on a gym crawl with grand-daughter Biljana—the gyms that had not closed for the summer, that is. The first place wasn't actually a gym but a room in a woman's house with the sign "Best Body Studio" above the door. Inside were two whiz-bang machines that resembled inverted male appendages called Power Plates. She explained how the machines worked.

"You get on this round platform and when you turn on the machine, the platform begins to vibrate. Stand with your feet apart in a squat and hold your stance for 30 seconds," she continued enthusiastically. "It's great for toning. Have a go."

She pushed Biljana and me onto the platform. I'm not sure about its efficacy with regard to toning, but I can guarantee it lets you know exactly what it is you *need* to tone—and a triple-support bra is mandatory.

The next gym was Belgrade's premier fitness centre. It had all the latest equipment (minus the Power Plates), plus pool, spa, sauna, lockers and regular aerobic exercise classes. Complimentary towels were provided, along with cotton buds and potpourri. The soles of my shoes were inspected and deemed appropriate for their polished floorboards. This was definitely the gym for me.

"How much for a month?"

"Nineteen-thousand dinar," replied the woman at the reception desk. This was equivalent to $270. I'd obviously misheard or she must have thought I meant a year. I repeated the question.

"Normally we don't allow memberships for under six months," she explained, "but since you're a visitor we'll make an exception and offer you one month at the special rate of 19 thousand dinar."

"Nineteen *hundred* dinar?" I politely queried.

"No, 19 *thousand* dinar." She was getting tetchy.

"But that's four times what I pay per month in Australia and more than three times what I paid in the US! You can't be serious!"

She was serious, so we headed to the next gym. It was only the size of half a tennis court, with a partition down the middle. On one side of the partition, the room was wall-to-wall and end-to-end crammed full of machinery, weights and barbells. I marvelled at how anyone managed to use the equipment because it overlapped with everything else. The other half of the room was littered with mats, bars and weight plates. I could have it all for the equivalent of just $40 per month. I took it, and had my first workout there and then.

I went to warm up on the rowing machine. I tried putting my feet in the straps, but there were no straps. I tried to select the resistance, but the resistance lever was broken. I looked for the display box, but there wasn't one. I informed the woman at the front desk.

"I know," she replied.

"When will it be fixed?" I queried.

"I don't know." She was not a forthcoming conversationalist.

On my second visit to the gym, I stepped onto the workout floor and instantly found myself skidding on my bottom from one end of the room to the other. I came to a stop at a pile of skipping ropes. The woman at the reception desk raised her head.

"Be careful. The floor's just been mopped." She returned to her magazine.

I was beginning to think the staircase at home might be my best option for a safe and affordable workout.

Irony

The world is but a canvas to our imaginations.
Henry David Thoreau

A few days after my crane-dodging jog, I plucked up the courage to go for a run in the other direction. After several perilous blocks, I was rewarded by arriving at the stalwart citadel of Kalemegdan. Perched on a ridge, the fortress overlooks the Great War Island and the confluence of the Sava and Danube Rivers. I paused to look at the winding waterways and grassy grandeur. A cool breeze brushed my cheeks and blew the complaining commentary out of my head. I was left standing in the present moment.

The late spring colours suddenly took on a new vividness, and my gaze swept across the picturesque parkland and eclectic towers, punctuated by fountains and statues. Facing the river was the notorious, nude Victory Monument, sculpted by Ivan Meštrović. The statue was meant to stand in the city centre but was banished to the grounds of the fortress on account of its nakedness. The Victor was surrounded by evidence of live concerts and young love.

But what impressed me most was a series of signs along the cliff edge, warning visitors: "Walking in this area you risk your life." I would have added: "On the contrary, walking in the *other* area you risk your life."

Beauty Secrets

What you see depends on what you're looking for.
Unknown

I asked cousin Milica the secret of her smooth skin.

"Cucumbers and egg yolks," she announced.

"Ingested or rubbed in?"

"Rubbed into the skin. Every time you slice up a cucumber, rub a piece all over your face and neck," she advised.

"And the egg yolk?" I squirmed.

"Separate it from the white and then coat your skin with it. Wait 10 minutes before washing it off, trying not to talk or move."

"She'll never last 10 minutes without opening her mouth," my father interjected.

Personal Touch

One of the diseases to afflict this century is a loss of wonder.
Madeleine L'Engle

Every morning, Milica's neighbour went to the local bakery and bought me a freshly baked, wholemeal, pumpkin-seed bread roll in the shape of a horseshoe—just because she'd overheard me say I liked them. It was always still warm to the touch when it arrived. Some days it was a bit burnt, some days it was a bit doughy, and other days it could be anywhere in between. I liked it precisely the way it came. I liked the fact that I never quite knew what it would be like. It reminded me that a real human being with conflicting demands had woken up much earlier than I had so that I could enjoy the product of their labour. It made me feel cared for.

Priorities

Teachers open the door, but you must enter by yourself.
Chinese proverb

Whatever anyone says about the Serbs, they do good dairy. The milk is good enough to drink straight and it's of two types only: normal fat and low fat. I found it a relief not to have more types and dozens of brands to choose from. Less choice meant much less time spent grocery shopping. The chocolate milk is liquid heaven, reminiscent of rich dark chocolate made fluid and kept in cold storage. The yoghurt is firm, refreshing and appropriately sour—the perfect accompaniment to the most flavoursome raspberries, blueberries and blackberries I've ever tasted.

The bearded old man at the markets selling berries always had a broad, toothy grin and allowed me to sample as many berries as I wanted while he weighed my purchase. The sampling stopwatch started from the time he placed the first shovelful on the scales and stopped when I told him to stop shovelling. There were two types of blueberries: smaller, darker, tangier wild blueberries, and larger, paler, sweeter "modified" blueberries, the latter more like the ones I was familiar with. Of course I had to buy both. The berry man never allowed me to buy too much at a time because he didn't want the berries to go off before I managed to eat them.

"I'm here every day, so you don't have to buy a whole week's worth in one visit. Come back and buy them fresh again tomorrow."

"But I might not have time to come tomorrow," I justified.

"How can you not have time for the important things in life?" he challenged. His observation was a timely wake-up call.

The woman in the next stall picked out the juiciest nectarines and apricots for me. Another visit to fruit heaven! I was permitted—in fact, encouraged—to try an apricot from each box, to make sure I bought the ones I liked.

Not long after, I discovered sun-dried capsicums.

"These are delicious," I smiled, paying for a bright red bundle tied with string.

"What do you stuff them with?" the proud grower asked.

"I don't stuff them; I munch on them just as they are."

"You're pulling my leg," he said. "In all my time I've never heard of anyone eating them raw. They're meant to be rehydrated, stuffed with minced meat and baked in the oven."

"I didn't know that. You should try them raw; they're great." He shook his head in disbelief.

That's when I saw the walnut women. Each guarded a large crate of fresh, crisp, caramel-coloured gems. I made a beeline for my brain-boosting friends.

"These are the best walnuts you'll ever taste," the wispier-haired woman announced. "Go ahead and try one." She was right.

"Now try mine," the second woman offered.

I frowned with mock solemnity. "I can't decide. I guess I'll have to buy half-a-kilogram from each of you."

"Walnuts are extremely good for your brain, heart and kidneys," the first woman divulged. "And if you eat a handful before bed, you'll get a good night's sleep." I hadn't known about the sleep benefits.

"During the NATO bombings of Yugoslavia in 1999, we couldn't keep up with the demand for walnuts. People were storing them in the event of a food shortage because they knew that walnuts were life-sustaining. They're very perishable, so you should put them in an airtight container and keep them in a cool, dry, dark place—they'll last for six months that way. You can also freeze them for up to a year."

I loved that every visit to the markets reinforced the dietary advice I'd been giving Dad. He never said anything, but hearing the same message from a neutral source—and his countrymen at that—would no doubt have made an impression on him.

I procured plums from the huge tree at the front of Milica's house. They were bright yellow and only the size of grapes but absolutely bursting with succulent sweetness. I had to balance on the head of the carved stone lion at Milica's doorstep to get to them. I soon picked everything I could reach, so one afternoon when the street was deserted, I took off my shoes and climbed onto the roof of a battered car parked in front of the house. I was having great success when I suddenly felt a burning sensation on the back of my legs. The car's owner had snuck up behind me and whacked me with a branch. I hurriedly slid down and mumbled an apology. But the plums were worth the whipping.

Support

*Here is the test to find whether your mission on earth is finished:
if you're alive, it isn't.*
Richard Bach

"There's a big difference between Milica's life and mine," Dad reflected soon after we'd arrived in Belgrade. "Even though she lost her husband 10 years ago, she'll always have a reason to live. She has two granddaughters to look after."

Milica's two hip-and-happening granddaughters didn't need looking after. Nevena, who was on university holidays, kept nocturnal hours and barely emerged for breakfast by dinner-time. Biljana popped in with her boyfriend every few days to check if Milica needed anything.

"It's not my job to give you grandchildren, so that you have a reason to live," I told Dad gently. "It's my role to support you in the choices *you* make to give your life meaning, purpose and fulfilment. Who's to say if you had grandchildren they wouldn't be off somewhere on the other side of the world, doing their own thing?

"You don't need to find an all-encompassing reason to live. If you make a positive difference to one person today, that's a reason to have lived today. You can figure out tomorrow's reason tomorrow. There will always be someone whose day you can brighten in some way—and that's a big deal. I know it's pointless telling you that you make a positive difference to *my* life, so I won't even go there. But just for the record, you do."

His look softened.

"Can't you see how happy you've made Milica by coming to see her?" I continued. "She's just beaming. She loves having you as a companion. And she's immensely grateful that you carry groceries and help her walk along that minefield of a street. She adores you and she loves fussing over you. But don't get used to it because it won't be happening when we get back to Sydney. I will not be peeling your eggs for you."

Listening

*To listen well is as powerful a means of influence
as to talk well.*
Chinese proverb

On the way home from the markets one sunny afternoon, Dad and I passed an old man sitting in front of a café with a newspaper. He was holding a magnifying glass to the page, trying to do a crossword. A wave of sadness unexpectedly washed over me.

About a block later, I noticed an optometrist. I pulled my father through the door, and confirmed with the receptionist that the optometrist was available. I then dragged Dad back to the old man with the magnifying glass.

"What are you doing?" Dad protested.

"We're going to get that old man some glasses, so he can do his crosswords without a magnifying glass."

We introduced ourselves to the man and spent the next hour listening to the old man's war stories. It turned out that he had macular degeneration, so glasses were of no use. But he was thrilled that we'd stopped to talk to him and he rewarded us with tales of intrigue, loyalty and narrow escapes. On resuming our walk, I turned to Dad with a smile.

"It's a good thing we're both alive today," I said. "We made a positive difference to that man."

Patience

As long as a man stands in his own way,
everything seems to be in his way.
Ralph Waldo Emerson

Out of the blue one morning, one of Dean's socks appeared among my father's laundry. Dean had been looking for it only a few days before we'd left Los Angeles. I decided it would be fun to return it to him with a postcard.

As soon as I entered the post office, I was assaulted by the shrill howls of a hysterical four-year-old child. The entire post office was only five metres square, and the place was reverberating with the racket. I'd been looking forward to a few minutes of respite from the clamour of construction work outside, but it wasn't to be. The boy was sitting in a chair, violently swinging his legs and rattling the seat in accompaniment to his wailing. I wondered why his parents weren't doing anything.

As I stood muttering gratitude for not having acquiesced to giving my father a grandchild, I observed a kind of operetta playing out. Everyone in the post office—both staff and customers—took it in turns to comfort the child. They joked, they stroked, they reassured, they appealed to his sense of "manhood", they caught his tears in a "magic tissue" and they asked him what could possibly be so distressing. No-one appeared to be annoyed, impatient or perturbed in any way. In a few minutes he settled down and was happily led out of the post office by his unruffled father. I was amazed and duly humbled.

When the boy had gone, the customers and staff resumed the sort of conversation I'd have with a girlfriend. They spoke about recent losses in their family, worrisome offspring, and how the rain had affected the quality of fruit and vegetables at the markets. Everything was within earshot. No-one in the queue seemed to mind this social exchange and when it was their turn, they did the same.

When it was *my* turn, I handed over an unsealed envelope containing the sock and the postcard, in case the contents needed to be inspected. "This is going to America," I said, ready to engage in banter about my travels.

"This isn't the counter for packages to America," I was told. "You have to go to the business counter."

"But this isn't business; it's going to a friend," I clarified.

"It doesn't matter. Packages to America are handled as business."

When I arrived at the correct counter and pulled out the sticky tape to seal the envelope, I was told that sticky tape was not permitted.

"Anyone could open the envelope and reseal it," the postal worker said, "without leaving a trace." She raised her eyebrows and lowered her chin.

I was about to launch into a why/wherefore/so what discussion but thought better of it. She applied Super Glue, not paper glue, to the envelope. I heaved a sigh of relief as I stepped back out into the dust and din of Belgrade.

I arrived back at Milica's house to discover that Dad had broken one of his denture teeth while sneaking a biscuit in my absence, so off we went to the nearest denturist. When we reached the address that Milica had scribbled on a piece of newspaper, Dad took one look at the dilapidated building and decided that he didn't want his tooth repaired in Serbia. He wanted to go to his tried and trusted denturist (my mate, Dennis) in Sydney. I didn't blame him, but I was concerned about more damage occurring if we left it.

"I'll be fine," he promised. "I'll look like one of the locals," he grinned.

Stalker

Strength does not come from physical capacity.
It comes from an indomitable will.
Mahatma Gandhi

After a week of contusions and lacerations sustained at the jumble yard that called itself a gym, I succumbed to joining Belgrade's Premier Fitness Centre. It was the best value $270 I've ever spent. The Serbs know how to treat their elite.

I hadn't realised there would be a personal trainer-cum-caddy at my beck and call. I had only so much as to drop my towel and someone would come *running* to pick it up. And would I prefer a fresh towel? Just a purposeful shake of my water bottle and it would be refilled for me. The slightest furrow of my brow brought a well-toned body and smiling face to my side, to ask how he could assist me. "And please, do treat your muscles to a warm pool or a hot spa when you've completed your workout. Here's a bigger towel for the purpose."

One evening, I arrived at the gym much later than usual and found only one other person in the weights room: a man who was well endowed and well aware of it (I'm referring to bulging biceps and cannonball calves, of course). It's not that I was deliberately looking; he was impossible to miss. After my warm-up on the rowing machine, I alternated between upper and lower body exercises. It quickly became apparent that as soon as I finished with a machine, my muscly companion would casually saunter over to it and use it himself, making a big show of having to adjust it to a much heavier weight. With all that testosterone and four times my muscle bulk, of course he'd be lifting at least triple what I was. After a while, his heaving, grunting and satisfied grinning started to irritate me. I know, I know—just breathe through it, but I was having enough trouble breathing through my workout.

So for my next exercise, I chose a machine that was directly behind him, so he wouldn't be able to see what I was doing. I completed my reps but this time added lots of sound effects. When I finished, I let out an almighty groan and before he could turn around, I silently adjusted the pin so the weight was 40 kilograms above what I'd actually been pushing. I then walked away from the machine and started stretching, as though I'd overdone it. True to form, he made straight for the machine I'd just left. He looked at the weight—then at me—then at the weight again. I worked very hard to keep a straight face. Not to be outdone by a puny female, he slowly withdrew the pin and placed it several notches beyond where I'd left it. He took a deep breath and began to push. The weights barely moved.

I made sure that he knew I was watching him adjust the weights back down, and I heard not a peep while he did his reps. I repeated my charade and performance—hissing, blowing and generally causing a ruckus—several more times before the end of my session. I laughed all the way home.

Rescue

There are more things, Lucilius, likely to frighten us than there are to crush us; we suffer more often in imagination than in reality.
From *Moral letters to Lucilius* by Seneca

Very early one morning, I was jolted awake by a rattling sound at the window. I pulled the covers over my head and tried to ignore it—noise at any time of day or night was one of Belgrade's trademarks. The more I tried to ignore it, the louder it became. Then the sound took on an urgent, unsettling clattering, followed by a heavy blow against the glass. I sat up. The scratching turned desperate and the entire window frame shook on its hinges.

Behind the curtains I saw the silhouette of a large, outspread hand banging against the pane. My pounding heart obscured the pounding on the glass. Someone was trying to break in! Was it the guy from the gym, seeking revenge? How could he hope to get in? The house had double windows and thick, iron window bars. Had I closed the windows properly? I scanned the room for a weapon. Antique plates, bowls, figurines, vases, lamps, books, picture frames, candleholders. A heavy bronze candelabrum! I could do considerable damage with it if I smashed it over the hand.

I slowly drew back the bedclothes and picked up the candelabrum with two hands. My heart was beating against my eardrums as I approached the window. The moment I raised my weapon, the sound subsided and the hand slid away from the pane, almost disappearing. I was suddenly startled by the meowing of a cat. So was the hand. It began its frenzied banging again. Then I realised. The hand was not a hand, but the wing of a frightened bird, taking refuge from the cat between the iron bars and the pane. My body shook with relief. I was breathing as though I'd just run a record sprint.

I pulled open the curtains just as the cat hurled itself against the bars. Poor little bird! How was I going to rescue it? If I opened the windows to let it inside, I'd never get it outside again. I did the only logical thing to do. I opened the two windows with the fly screens so the bird was still unable to get in. I then hid myself from view of the cat and began barking, punctuated with vicious, blood-curling growls and snarls! Both animals froze, and then the cat withdrew.

"Quick! Fly away before the cat comes back," I urged the bird. She sat there nursing her own pounding heart.

Unfortunately, all the barking had woken my father.

"What's going on in here?" he said, bursting into the room.

"Sorry, I'd forgotten you were asleep. I was just scaring a cat away."

"Have you gone nuts? You scared the living daylights out of *me*, never mind some cat!"

"It was trying to kill this bird."

"Is there any chance you might settle back down and go to sleep? Or at least let *me* sleep?"

"Sure, just as soon as I'm certain the bird is safe."

In a moment of apparent comprehension, the bird slipped out between the bars and flew away.

Sharing

*Thousands of candles can be lit from a single candle,
and the life of the candle will not be shortened.
Happiness never decreases by being shared.*
Buddha

Biljana and her boyfriend, Milan, took us to Serbia's largest Orthodox Church, Sveti (Saint) Sava, named after the founder of the independent Serbian Orthodox religion. At night it was beautifully lit, with massive, white, luminous domes dominating the city skyline from many miles away. It began life as a small church in 1895 and is still a work in progress, financed entirely by donations. It took 40 days just to lift the 4 000 tonne dome into place.

Dad was born in a small apartment not far from Sveti Sava, to parents Mira and Michael. He was delivered by a midwife at home, and soon after, the family moved into a larger house. Michael had a degree in chemistry and worked as a teacher in a local private school; he had two brothers, also teachers, one of whom was Milica's father. Mira, the youngest of seven children, was reputed to be exceptionally beautiful. My father was the younger of two sons. His tall, tousle-haired brother, Branko, was two-and-a-half years his senior.

In the streets behind the church we came to a chic, bohemian café called Maska (meaning *mask*). It was in an elegant, three-storey mansion with indoor and outdoor seating and a smoky ambience. As our group waited for drinks, I wandered inside to have a look around. The lighting on each floor became dimmer the higher I climbed. The bar stools were carved in the shape of cupped hands: the broad, flat palm formed the seat, and the fingers curled up to provide a back support. The top floor had dark, angled couches surrounded by antiques and overhanging plants. It was the perfect setting for sneaking furtive kisses in the shadows; the colourful paraphernalia would discreetly obscure any waywardness. I was suddenly struck by a subtle pang of longing—the yearning to share this experience with an intimate other.

Revolving Door

*Life's challenges are not supposed to paralyse you; they're
supposed to help you discover who you are.*
Bernice Johnson Reagon

After our visit to Sveti Sava, Dad was keen to see the house where
he'd spent most of his childhood and early adulthood. Milan and
Biljana drove us there; my father had no trouble remembering
the location. The house had been sold decades ago, after Dad's
mother had died in a residential care facility. She was described
as having "lost it"; her symptoms sounded like Alzheimer's
Disease.

"This is where you spent the first year of your life," my father
announced as we arrived. The building was largely obscured
by a tall stone wall and a grand, old oak tree, but I could spy
elaborate stonework and elegant arches.

"Mira, my mother, lived with us and she was very possessive of
you," my father recalled. "But when you were one year old, she
gave me an ultimatum: if I didn't divorce my wife, she'd throw
us out of the house. I didn't wait for her to throw us out. We left
the very next day."

I was intrigued to hear more, but Dad was already returning
to the car. "The new owner has made a lot of alterations to the
facade," he remarked, abruptly changing the subject. A few blocks
away, we stopped in front of another house. "This was the home
of your godparents, who took us in when we left my mother's
house." He was pointing to a much smaller, simpler building.
"Your godparents were retired and had no children of their own,
so they delighted in looking after you, while your mum and I
went to work. After a year, your maternal grandparents decided
it was their turn to look after you, so you went to live with them

in Vršac, about two hours' bus ride from Belgrade. Your mother and I stayed in Belgrade because of work, but we visited you as often as we could on weekends. After a year, we brought you back to Belgrade to live with your godparents again."

I was amazed at my own story. "Didn't I object to this revolving door system of care?"

"Of course you did. You howled when we took you away from your godparents the first time. And you howled when we took you away from your maternal grandparents. And you howled when we took you away from your godparents the second time in order to come to Australia. But you adjusted very quickly because you were always in a loving environment. We were lucky to find a kind Serbian woman in Australia, who took care of you in the first year after our arrival. Then we brought your maternal grandparents out, and all of us lived under the same roof, so we didn't need a nanny any more."

A hypothesis took shape in my mind. As a baby, I never learnt that long-term bonds were possible. Loving, close relationships all ended in painful, inevitable separation. As a child, I was divorced from my primary care-giver each year and handed to someone else. Did this establish a blueprint, whereby I instinctively shied away from commitment and long-term relationships? Was it a coincidence that my 25-year pattern of serial monogamy reflected my earliest years? I'd always had loving boyfriends, but after a few years I consistently experienced a nagging sense that "something wasn't right" and I ended up leaving the relationship. I still felt warmly about my ex-partners, and after the obligatory year of emotional havoc that followed a break up, we became friends. But it was a pattern I was growing tired of.

How to break out of it? Was awareness enough? Since the brain is plastic, I knew it was possible to rewire myself and unlink love from inescapable demise. But how? And was this really the case, or was my self-diagnosis just an indulgent excuse for fickleness?

Pin-Up Girl

You are never too old to set another goal
or to dream a new dream.
C. S. Lewis

It was the evening of 19 July. Dad and I were going out to dinner, to meet one of Mum's closest girlfriends, Danica. As a child, Danica lived a long way from the local school, so when she was 10 years old she came to live with my mother's family, who lived much closer to the school. Mum was an only child, then seven years old. The two girls struck an immediate bond that lasted for the duration of my mother's life. They were like sisters.

When I stepped out of my room wearing black-and-white checked shorts and my Empire State Building T-shirt, my father was not impressed. "You're not going out dressed like that. Put on a skirt and some nice sandals. Show a bit of respect."

"Everyone dresses like this."

"Not when they're meeting an elderly lady for the first time. I won't have it."

I knew better than to stand my ground and have him sulking the entire evening. Since we were catching a trolleybus (a cross between a tram and a bus) from Milica's house to Trg Republike (Republic Square), it didn't matter that my sandals were giving me blisters.

After one stop, a 10 year-old boy hopped on the trolleybus and proceeded to cruise up and down the aisle, singing. Loudly. Stridently. Shrilly. Over-enthusiastically. Mock-operatically. Mournfully. All the while holding a tatty, malodorous cap under the nose of each passenger until they were forced to throw in a coin because they could no longer hold their breath. Just as I was about to ask how much I'd need to pay him to *stop* singing, the trolleybus came to a halt a full two kilometres from our destination.

"Everyone disembark here please," the driver called out. "The police are preventing public vehicles from entering the city centre."

"What's the problem?" I asked.

"Croatian President Josipović is visiting Belgrade to speak to President Tadić."

"But I thought they had their talks yesterday."

"It seems they got on so well they're still gasbagging."

Normally I would have skipped those two kilometres but I knew my feet would be skinless after a few hundred metres in my sandals.

"I'm going to take off my sandals," I told Dad.

"Not on your life," he said. "We'll walk slowly. We're not in a hurry."

By the time we met Danica, the tops of my toes looked like a lawn mower had run over them. I was in so much pain, I could hardly spit out a greeting.

"I've heard you don't mind walking," chirped Danica, "so I'm taking you to a traditional Serbian restaurant opposite the citadel. It's about a kilometre from here but well worth the effort."

"That sounds perfect," replied my father.

I felt a deep commiserative bond with all the mothers I'd heard complaining about their five-year-olds: "He's such a terror at home but when we're out, people think he's an angel." If *I'd* suggested walking a kilometre to a restaurant, Dad would have flatly refused. But tonight, when each step was an excursion into hell, he could think of nothing more pleasant than walking. At the first café, I excused myself and found the bathroom. I grabbed great wads of toilet paper and stuffed them underneath my sandal straps. What a relief.

When we reached the restaurant, Danica went to greet the manager and Dad and I reviewed the menu.

"I might just go straight to dessert," my father nonchalantly remarked. "My dentures have become really loose and they're hurting. I don't think I can chew anything, so I'll have to go for the vanilla custard slice or a plate of ice-cream."

"Or the bean soup," I suggested. I was struggling to maintain composure. "Why didn't you mention your denture problems earlier? Or were you planning to subsist on ice-cream for the next three weeks?"

"Don't make everything into such a big deal. I'm fine with soft foods like kajmak (a dairy product containing 60 per cent milk fat) and ajvar (red capsicum relish). And, of course, ice-cream. The weather's been so hot, the only sensible thing to eat is ice-cream."

"Tomorrow we're going to the denturist, first thing in the morning," I declared. "It isn't just about the ice-cream; it's about your dental health and hygiene."

Danica's return to the table interrupted our exchange. I enjoyed the evening more than I'd anticipated. She was a sprightly, engaging and candid 74 year-old, who walked five kilometres every morning and refused to let old age dictate her life. She was the role model I'd been looking for. I wanted to jump up and hug her.

"I'm sick of everyone talking about their long-sightedness," she began. "A far bigger problem is our psychological *short*-sightedness.

"I can't deny that loss accompanies ageing. But it also brings a sense of security about who you are and what's really important. When I was young, I walked around as though I had a veil in front of my eyes. Getting old has given me the courage to rip off the veil and see the world as it really is. I'm no longer swayed by other people's values and judgements because I feel I've had enough experience to decide for myself. I'm much less fearful because I've proved that whatever life throws my way, I'll be able to handle it. And I ask more questions and have deeper conversations now than before because I'm not afraid of being emotionally overwhelmed.

"I think it's madness that young people try to defy ageing. All that botox, lasers, imported Russian hormones and gravity-defying breasts won't change your date of birth," she chuckled. "If women spent half the time exercising that they spent worrying about beauty products, they'd look a whole lot younger without *needing* beauty products! I watch my granddaughters spend hours talking about make-up, experimenting with make-up, choosing make-up and swapping make-up. Yet when I ask them about physical exercise, they tell me they don't have time!"

I wanted this woman as my pin-up girl.

"Correct me if I'm wrong," Danica continued, "but my doctor tells me that my daily walk keeps me off cholesterol medication and keeps me mentally switched on. Not to mention that it's improved my sex life!" She winked. "But that's probably too much information."

"Not at all," I said. "That's exactly what I've been telling Dad for the last six months, but he doesn't believe me. He prefers to think I'm a sadist."

"Oh, no!" she turned to my father. "As long as you're on this earth, you have to make the most of it. You owe it to God because He's keeping you here for a reason. And you owe it to your dear wife because she worked hard to create the best possible life for all three of you. It'll honour her if you live in the spirit in which she lived, giving generously to others in any way she could. As long as we're alive, we have the capacity to give—even if it's just a smile. The alternative to giving is being miserable. Making the effort is the cure for misery. As long as you're striving to do something or to get somewhere, you're on the right track, whatever that track might be." She paused for permission to continue.

"I can't imagine how much it hurts to have lost the dearest person in your life. I get upset every time I remember that I'll never speak to her again, and it must be a hundred-fold harder for you. But I've found that after a major loss, we need to learn new ways to appreciate life. We need to focus on small, daily miracles and to invent ways of creating our own. Sorry—I'm rambling, I talk too much."

"No, please keep going," I encouraged.

"This may sound strange, but I don't think there's anything inherently better about being 25 than 75. It's simply different. My granddaughters look forward with anticipation, and I look back with contentment—and I can still look forward with anticipation. I'm by no means ready to die, but I'm also not afraid to die because I know I've lived. I've given it my best shot. I have no regrets."

Back Track

*Slow down and everything you are chasing will come around
and catch you.*
John De Paola

"Where's my tooth?" Dad wailed.

"What tooth?" I was still bleary-eyed and half asleep.

"The tooth that broke off my denture the other day." It was futile asking him where he last saw it.

"I'm sure we'll find it," I replied. "I'll help you look."

"I'm so useless. I'm always losing things," he moaned.

"Just because we didn't bring our 'Can Do' jars to Belgrade doesn't mean the rules of the game don't apply. Putting yourself down is still off limits. And it isn't true. You're extremely useful and you always find things in the end."

"Maybe I dropped it."

The carpet was of long, shaggy, cream-coloured pile—the perfect camouflage for a tooth. We combed every fibre and carefully inspected every surface in his room and bathroom. Every five minutes of searching pushed Dad's distress level one notch higher.

"Tell me something," I asked in my most calm and soothing voice, "if you were going to put your tooth somewhere very safe, where would you put it?"

"In a glass of water by the bed," he responded instantly.

"OK, it's not there, so let's go back one step further. Where would you get the glass of water?"

"From the kitchenette."

Sure enough, there was a glass of water containing a tooth behind the tap in the kitchenette. We immediately set off for Belgrade's most reputable denture maker—not the same place we'd been to a week earlier. The first visit involved a lot of gagging and mould-making. The second visit, a day later, was to collect the fruits of her labour.

I was very impressed with the technician's work and patience. Within 24 hours, she had re-attached the broken tooth, as well as built up the base of the denture so it would sit comfortably in my father's mouth. When he first inserted it, he said it felt OK but the left side was rubbing. So she shaved a piece off the left edge. When he inserted it the second time, he said it felt OK but the right side was rubbing. So she shaved a piece off the right edge. When he placed it in his mouth the third time, he said there was a slight tinge on the left side again. She said to give it a few days to settle in and then reassess how it felt. If we needed to, we could come back any time and she'd adjust it free of charge.

After a hearty Serbian meal—what other kind of Serbian meal is there?—and an uninterrupted sleep, the dentures settled in perfectly.

Joy

Tension is who you think you should be.
Relaxation is who you are.
Chinese proverb

It all happened the day I discovered the sweetest, juiciest blackberries on the planet. The taste exploded out of them. I'd probably eaten an ice-cream container-full by the time I arrived home and was contemplating heading straight back out to buy more. But first I had to use the bathroom.

I slipped into the secluded little bathroom in the hallway, that no-one ever used. As I turned the doorknob to exit the bathroom, it came off in my hand. I tried to reattach it but had no success. I gently pushed the door. It refused to budge. I forcefully pushed the door. It remained immovable. I knocked in the vain hope that someone would hear. There was no reply. The knocking turned to banging and then shouting. No-one was likely to walk past unless they were leaving the house. I had no mobile phone. Dad would assume I'd gone for a walk or taken myself to the gym. I was trapped. I was not happy. I was sick of this cumbrance of a house.

I decided to meditate. I sat down on the toilet lid and closed my eyes. This is ridiculous, I thought. At least if I had a book … Maybe if I banged on the back wall … Why do these things always happen to me? What is life trying to tell me? Why am I having this conversation in my head? I'm supposed to be pressing the pause button on my thinking. This is supposed to be calming me down, not getting me worked up. This is a perfect opportunity for meditation and I'm wasting it …

My internal babble continued. I eventually opened my eyes to stop the noise in my head and I saw a curious object. It was a figurine of an ape in a contemplative pose, holding a human skull—not what I'd associate with a bathroom. The ape was sitting on a pile of books, one of which had *Darwin* etched on its spine. The ape and the skull stared at each other, and *I* stared at them. After a while, I realised I'd been looking without thinking. My internal racket had subsided and I felt serene. There was stillness, both within and without. It was delicious. I started giggling—I was enjoying just *being*. Was I going mad? Either that or I'd discovered the meaning of life. It was a pleasure just to breathe … to look … to listen … to be aware. I had never experienced anything like it. I was happy for no reason.

My breathing fascinated me. I followed each breath, trying to catch the moment between in and out. I was deeply rooted in the present moment and life was beautiful. I felt a heightened sense of awareness—colours seemed brighter, sounds seemed sharper. Imprisoned in a bathroom with nothing to do, I felt freer and happier than I had ever felt.

I suddenly understood—*really* understood—what Sarah had said on the day of my meltdown back in Sydney. My big lesson was to learn to *accept* my father, not mould him.

I had always shunned the word "acceptance" because I equated it with passivity, inertia, apathy, defeatism and resignation. In contrast, I valued action, determination, persistence and perseverance. But now it dawned on me that acceptance didn't negate action, if action was required. Acceptance wasn't about giving up or putting up with an intolerable situation. It was about recognising that everything was part of a bigger picture, one that I wasn't always privy to. Acceptance was about not making assumptions or jumping to conclusions. Acceptance was about remembering that I was sitting on a train, looking out a window, and only able to see what was directly in front of me. I was unable to see the view from anyone else's window. And Dad was in a different seat, looking out a different window. I had never seen what he had seen, nor could I ever know what he was seeing.

At that moment I heard voices. "Hey!" I called out. "Open the door! The door knob broke off and I can't get out!" Dad had to remove the door from its hinges to let me out.

"This could only ever happen to you," he shook his head.

"Thanks," I said. "You're my hero."

As we prepared for bed that night, I asked my father a seemingly random question. I had no agenda or preconceived idea about where it might lead.

"Dad, what's the most important thing in life?"

He thought about it briefly. "Love. Without a doubt, it's love. What could be more important, more valuable, more comforting or more beautiful than feeling a warm glow about someone and knowing that they reciprocate? Knowing that someone deeply cares about you is the foundation for everything else. Having someone with you as you ride the ups and downs of life makes the unbearable somehow bearable. That constancy helps you to keep your head above water.

"It's the disintegration of love that's responsible for all the chaos in the world. Fractured families lead to insecurity and lack of trust. And insecurity makes people do rash and cruel things. People who are hurting inflict hurt. Love washes away the inclination to be unkind to others."

He turned to me with moist eyes. "What's the most important thing for a newborn child?"

"Love," I replied.

"I never had that. My mother never loved me. She was incapable of loving anyone but herself."

Dad then told me his story.

In His Words

Listening is a magnetic and strange thing, a creative force. The friends who listen to us are the ones we move toward. When we are listened to, it creates us, makes us unfold and expand.
Brenda Ueland

My earliest memory is that of lying in bed next to my brother, Branko. We were supposed to be taking an afternoon nap. A stunning, angelic-looking woman with thick, dark hair, wearing a flowing white dress, entered the house. My father turned to look at her without speaking. As she approached, I pretended to be asleep. She kissed both of us and left without saying a word.

My mother, Mira, could never settle for "ordinary". My father, Michael, had courted her for years but he knew that to win her, he had to stand out as someone "special". So he borrowed a large sum of money and bought a car, an elitist rarity in those days. Mira was duly impressed and married him. The moment she fell pregnant with my brother, Michael sold the car and repaid his debt. Mira was furious. Two years later, she became pregnant with me and tried to procure an abortion. The doctors refused because they needed the consent of both parents and my father wouldn't hear of it.

When I was exactly one year and six days old, my mother left my father and went to live with her sister, Vesna, who was 15 years her senior. Vesna was happily married but unable to have children. When Mira arrived with my brother and me, Vesna's husband said she could stay if she took us children back to Michael. Without hesitation, Mira went straight to Michael's workplace and deposited a child into each arm. Michael couldn't look after us on his own, so he left us with his parents. Thereafter, Mira occasionally came to visit.

About two years later, Michael surreptitiously organised for his mother, who was Bulgarian, to take us to Bulgaria. No-one was to know, and Michael made clandestine plans to leave Yugoslavia himself. One day, Mira found an empty house when she came to visit. She asked everyone in the neighbourhood where we were, but no-one could help her. After a few weeks, she began receiving postcards: *The children and I are holidaying in Vienna... The children and I are loving Paris.*

Then the postcards abruptly stopped, to be replaced by rumours—Michael had murdered us and was living in self-imposed exile in Naples. Or maybe Milan. Police in Austria and France were notified to look for a dark-haired man with two small boys. A reward was offered. After 18 months of searching, a cleaning lady presented to the Yugoslav authorities and said she'd overheard Michael mention Sofia, capital of Bulgaria, shortly before his disappearance.

My mother and her brother, Želko, went straight to the Bulgarian embassy in Belgrade. She had no trouble engaging the authorities to assist her—her attractiveness and her alluring manner ensured that she always got her way. The Bulgarian consul promised Mira he'd have news for her within three weeks. Sure enough, Mira received word that an elderly woman and two young boys were living in a small house near the foot of Mount Vitosha. The children matched Mira's description, but someone needed to go to Bulgaria to identify them. Boys were potential Bulgarian soldiers, and the nation was reluctant to relinquish them; girls would have been handed over more readily.

A covert operation was organised. A soccer match and cycling race were arranged between Yugoslavia and Bulgaria. Among the cyclists were undercover policemen, and linesmen from both countries were employed for the soccer match—among them, my Uncle Želko. The police took Uncle Želko to the house on the edge of Sofia as soon as the match was over.

When they arrived, Branko and I were playing outside. I was pulling apart a crate. Uncle Želko called out to me. I looked up but didn't recognise him, so I continued with my game. But Branko remembered our uncle and cried out his name. It was all the proof the authorities needed. At the divorce settlement three years previously, I'd been consigned to the care of my mother, while Branko had been assigned to my father. Therefore my mother could only lay claim to me, not to Branko. I was snatched from my crate, bundled into a car and driven to the Yugoslav consulate in Sofia. I remember shrieking and struggling to get free. I was four-and-a-half years old.

At the consulate, I was ordered to wait quietly in a large, sparsely furnished room. The door handle was too high for me to reach, but I managed to drag a chair to the door and open it. I saw my grandmother and Branko speaking to some men in uniform. I cried out and was immediately seized by a big, hairy arm and returned to the room. The chair was removed and I spent the night at the consulate. I wet the bed. I spent several more nights at the consulate and wet the bed every night—and for many months thereafter. It must have been Christmas time because in the building's foyer was a Christmas tree with a red, battery-operated toy train circling it.

Eventually, Uncle Želko and I returned to Belgrade by train with a Yugoslav policeman sent to accompany us. Uncle Želko tried to sleep, but I kept pulling the pillow from under his head and waking him up. My mother was waiting at the station in Belgrade. Uncle Želko lifted me above his head, to show Mira he had fulfilled his mission.

Mira looked at him and scowled. "I don't want *him*. I want Branko."

*****

Not long after, Branko and my grandmother were also deported back to Yugoslavia because we'd all been living in Bulgaria illegally. They went to live with my father's brothers because my father was nowhere to be found—later we discovered that he had escaped to Bolivia. Mira tried to exchange me for Branko, but the courts wouldn't allow it. Eventually, Aunt Vesna managed to convince her to give up the fight and accept the son she'd been given.

Vesna's husband had since died, so I grew up with my mother, aunt and maternal grandmother. Mira ruled the roost because she had the most volatile temperament, never backed down on anything and was adored by her sister. Aunt Vesna essentially raised me, and it seemed the more my mother hated me, the more Vesna loved me. As for my grandmother, I remember her as a kind, soft, bulky woman, who always wore grey. She died at the age of 72.

In contrast, Mira would beat me. She used a thick stick or a thin stick, applied to my back or buttocks, depending on the severity of my offence. Sometimes I think she just felt like hitting me because I was there.

Very occasionally, I earned the right to kiss my mother. All I ever wanted was for her to love me.

On the rare occasions that Mira was without a chaperone, she would take me with her to meet her friends or go to the cinema. If we ever encountered one of *my* friends, they'd blurt out, "Wow, how come you never told us you had such a gorgeous girlfriend!" Mira loved it.

I landed in gaol about half a dozen times as a teenager. Most of the charges were spurious—the main reason was that we were classified as bourgeois—but one time it was my fault. My best friend, Jovan, and I sat next to each other at school every day for eight years. We were always mucking around and told each other everything. One day, I confided in Jovan that my mother had an Italian lover who wanted to take us to Italy. It was illegal for us to leave the country, so it was all being arranged secretly. Jovan reported us to the authorities, and both Mira and I were interrogated and imprisoned.

My mother also spent frequent bouts in prison. The longest time was 12 months. I was 16 at the time and went to stay with Aunt Vesna, who had remarried and was no longer living with us. My mother's crime had been to harbour a political prisoner in her basement for several months. When he received a radio one day, officials picked up the signals and traced them to our house. He'd fled, leaving Mira to pay the penalty. Throughout the year I went to visit her in prison. One evening, the weather was so bad I couldn't return home and had to spend the night in an all-female cell with her. I'd never heard such foul language in all my life.

When I was 18, Mira allowed me to go to my first Popovic Slava. Slava is the feast day of a Serbian Orthodox family patron saint. Each family has its own saint and therefore celebrates Slava on a different day. Mira's refusal to let me attend a Popovic Slava had been a statement of contempt towards my father's family. When I arrived, one of my father's brothers bounded over and asked, "Do I remind you of anyone?"

"No," I answered.

"Don't you think I'm the spitting image of your father?"

"I don't know," I replied. "I've never seen my father."

Ironically, Mira never knew her own father because he died six months before she was born. Mira's mother didn't want the new baby, so she stopped feeding her at four months, hoping that Mira would die. Mira's sister, Vesna, discovered what her mother was doing and threatened to report her to the police—from then on, Vesna took care of Mira. Vesna's affection for Mira became all the stronger when she discovered that she couldn't have children of her own. Mira was beautiful from a very young age and remained so all her life. When she was three years old, an Austrian diplomat and his wife offered the family a large sum of money to adopt her. Vesna vehemently refused.

I guess one thing I can thank my mother for was that her hurtfulness sent us to Australia. Your mum had badgered me to migrate to Australia from the day we met, but I told her I'd never leave Yugoslavia while my mother was alive. I had promised myself that I would never abandon Mira, despite being forced out of her house. I wanted to be there if she ever needed me. One day, not long after your second birthday, Helena, I ran into my mother at the train station. I hadn't seen her for several months. I asked how she was going.

"You don't care how I'm going," she snarled. "All you care about is your inheritance."

*****

Dad broke down at this point and we both cried.

"Your mother never knew a mother's love either," I offered through my tears.

"But at least she had a sister's love. I had no-one. Even though Vesna loved me, I didn't have regular access to her. I had snatches of love. It wasn't enough. What my mother said to me at the station that day was the final straw. I went straight home and told your mum to make plans for Australia."

Fragments

You may think that you have nothing worth giving,
that you have nothing remarkable to contribute, that you are
insignificant to the big picture. This would be a tragic mistake.
Harry M. Miller

Dad's chronicle overwhelmed me. I realised I'd been trying to reassemble a jigsaw, 79 years in the making, only to find I'd been missing the most important pieces. The pain and sadness in his eyes stretched back to a place I could never reach. His self-doubt, hesitation and apprehension took on a discernible shape. They formed a solid tree with deep roots and extensive branches, hung with behaviours I so readily dismissed as inertia, laziness and stubbornness. I was ashamed of all my self-serving assumptions and judgements. My limited interpretation of his outlook and conduct was a self-erected barrier to compassion and understanding.

Dad's story was the filter through which he experienced life. It was far more disabling than his dementia and far more entrenched. He still saw the world through the eyes of an unloved, little boy. Every time I thought about it, I choked up. He was still under the spell of a mother who herself had been under the same spell. As they saw it, both were born into a world that didn't want them; both were alive by default.

I tried to encourage Dad. "The fact that you were born, in spite of your mother's misgivings, means that *life itself* wanted you," I said, but even as I formed the words, I knew they wouldn't break the spell. The only wand I could wave was silent, unconditional acceptance. That word—acceptance—kept reverberating in my mind.

Birthday

Death is a reminder that we are alive.
Unknown

It was Dad's birthday, and Milica, Biljana and Milan were taking us to dinner at what they described as "one of the most health-conscious and sophisticated restaurants in Belgrade", overlooking the Sava River. It had a stylish, modern décor and extensive "European Fusion" menu. I liked what I saw.

After considerable deliberation, I selected the tuna steak, on the rare side. It was accompanied by a light salad of mixed greens and cherry tomatoes. I also ordered a side of sautéed vegetables, even though it was not on the menu. "No problem," replied our waiter.

One thing I very much liked about Serbian eateries of any size was that they didn't mind my habit of deconstructing the menu. This practice alternately embarrassed, infuriated or tried the patience of whoever I dined with. My logic was: why couldn't I mix and match the main feature of one dish with the accompaniment listed for another? Or ask for ingredients to be omitted that didn't appeal to my palate or principles? I didn't see any harm in asking. If the answer was no, so be it.

Everyone's meal was exquisitely presented and tasted superb. I beamed with contentment. I was so happy that Dad was spending his birthday with his all-time favourite relative in relaxing, beautiful surrounds. I'd wondered whether his first birthday without Mum might be a sad occasion for him, but he looked to be enjoying himself.

The only thing nagging me was the escalating heat. Everyone else was wearing a cardigan or jumper, yet I was ready to explode out of my skin. I felt flushed, my eyes were irritating me and I was developing a headache. I struggled to get through my meal and excused myself to go to the bathroom. By the time I got there, I was ready to faint. My pulse was racing and my heart wanted to burst. My skin was being overtaken by red, raised, urticarial weals, spreading by the second. I was simultaneously nauseous and wanting to open my bowels.

Surely I wasn't having an anaphylactic reaction? I didn't want to disrupt Dad's birthday—the cake was about to arrive, and everyone was waiting for me to light the candles—but I needed urgent medical attention. It would ruin things if I died on my father's birthday. As it was, I lasted until he blew out the candles. Then with feigned calm I announced, "Do you mind if we eat the cake at home? I need you to take me to a doctor."

"You *are* a doctor," Dad reminded me.

But Biljana had noticed my face. "Are you feeling OK? You're all flushed and your eyes are watering."

"I just need some medication—quickly."

"Can we take you to a chemist? It's Sunday afternoon and the hospital emergency department will be chaos."

"A hospital," I croaked. I wanted an injection of adrenaline before my throat began to swell and compromise my breathing. Dad became concerned.

"Are you sick? What's the matter?"

"I'm having an allergic reaction to something."

"But you're not allergic to anything."

"I am now."

"There's a chemist nearby. We can get some antihistamines for you."

"I need something a bit stronger than antihistamines." Antihistamines might relieve my intensely itchy rash but wouldn't help with life-threatening anaphylaxis.

"But I ordered exactly the same meal as you did," commented Milica.

"This isn't food poisoning. The food was fine but it contained something that's set off a severe allergic reaction throughout my entire body."

Everything seemed to occur in slow motion. It took an inordinate amount of time to get the bill. Then the restaurant didn't have the correct change. In the end they returned some of our money and said they trusted us to bring back what we owed them! While this was happening, I asked for a list of the ingredients in my meal, but no culprit emerged.

The traffic was diabolical. I was squeezed in the back seat, feeling dizzy and light-headed. I had no muscle tone and was immensely drowsy; I might have even fainted. I was jolted awake by the car hurtling onto the footpath.

"There's nowhere to park and the hospital is still miles away, so let's at least buy some antihistamines," said Milan.

The cold night air smacked me in the face and I felt somewhat revived. Fifteen minutes later, antihistamines on board, we were heading home. My rash was already fading and I felt I was out of danger. It was possible that my own endogenous adrenaline had kicked in and saved the day. I slept soundly for 12 hours and haven't been anywhere without an EpiPen since.

Whirlwind

*Learn everything you can, anytime you can, from anyone you
can; there will always come a time when
you will be grateful you did.*
Sarah Caldwell

When Milica's daughter, Gorica, arrived from Moscow for a few days, she took us on a whirlwind tour of Belgrade. We saw the fascinating Royal Compound, residence of the royal family; the villas and mansions of prestigious Dedinje; Maršal Tito's grave; Ada Ciganlija, an extremely popular recreational island in the Sava River; Košutnjak Park and its "health path", a socialist government initiative to foster a fit and able-bodied nation; a boat cruise on the Danube; street music in cobble-stoned, bohemian Skadarska; high tea at the Hyatt Hotel and more restaurants and cafés in a day than I'd conceive of covering in a week. I loved it.

I was growing to love Belgrade's inconsistencies and eclecticism. Sushi bars alternate with dimly lit dens and pastel-coloured, neo-Renaissance architecture. Untouched remnants of the 1999 bombings stand alongside newly renovated government buildings. Flamboyant bars, elegant patisseries, lurid discos, upmarket Italian restaurants, barbequed corn stalls, buzzing cafés, old-fashioned popcorn stands and street corner toy vendors all happily combine to form a colourful, vibrant, enticing scene. I even stumbled across the odd tofu supplier and macrobiotic wholefood outlet. Modern life was banging at Belgrade's door.

The city kept my kind of hours. Dinner was served until 1 am, corner stores never closed before 10 pm, and just down the road was a friendly 24-hour supermarket. I enjoyed that by the end of every taxi ride the driver felt like my best friend. I speak Serbian with a faint Australian accent, which kept them guessing where I was from.

Dad was intrigued by how much Belgrade had changed in 30 years. His long-term memory was largely intact, which boosted his confidence and confirmed to him that his faculties of recollection were still working. Short-term memory formation was a whole different ballgame, but the important thing was for him to focus on what was working.

Overseas travel is a massive brain booster. Fresh sights, sounds, scents and tastes stimulate our senses. The unfamiliarity and the break from routine force us to pay attention to our surroundings much more than usual. We're constantly meeting new people, contending with different ways of doing things and dealing with daily challenges. We tend to engage in more incidental exercise. We often speak in a foreign language or at least find creative ways to express ourselves. In short, we're more mindful and in perpetual learning mode and our brains are flourishing.

Divine Retribution

Sometimes we stare so long at a door that is closing that we see too late the one that is open.
Alexander Graham Bell

Dad and I were catching a bus to Novi Sad to spend two days with my grandmother's brother's widow. Novi Sad is the atmospheric and attractive capital city of Vojvodina, 90 minutes northwest of Belgrade.

We bought return tickets and also received metal tokens to allow us through the turnstile onto the bus platform. Dad wanted his token and bus ticket. I refused to give them to him because I knew he'd either lose them or put them somewhere so "safe" that we wouldn't find them for two days. I didn't tell him this—that would be negative programming—so I simply slipped them into my pocket and told him I'd prefer to keep everything together. He objected. I stood my ground. We argued. I refused to budge and took myself to the bathroom to get away from him.

They were the first crouch toilets I'd encountered in the country. I was momentarily confused about which way to face but I managed to place my feet in the appropriate grooves and promptly dropped my pants. Then I heard a clinking sound followed by a faint plop. I looked down to see our turnstile tokens disappear into a brown, bottomless pit. I froze in disbelief. Had this been the usual sit-down toilet, I could have—with a lot of psyching up—retrieved them by hand. But those tokens were already in the bowels of the earth. They weren't coming back, so I took a deep breath (which I immediately regretted), finished my business and stepped back out into the sunlight.

I felt sick, not because I'd need an official to unlock a gate to let us onto the platform, but because I'd refused to give Dad his token. I still had the bus tickets, so I knew we'd be allowed onto the bus. The issue was my father's reaction. My first thought was to sneak out of the bathroom without him noticing, so I could surreptitiously get replacement tokens. But he was right there as I emerged.

"Let's go and reserve a seat," he urged. "The bus has arrived at the platform."

"Sure. I just have to speak to someone first."

"Who?"

"Just wait," I ordered.

"Why? What's wrong?"

I spotted a nice young man in uniform and ran to explain our plight. He raised his eyebrows, checked our tickets and allowed us through the side gate with a smirk.

"What was that all about?" asked my father when we were on the bus. "Why didn't you use the tokens?"

I shrugged.

"You lost them!" He broke into a grin. "After not letting me have mine, you go and lose them! How?"

"Down the toilet."

He laughed almost all the way to Novi Sad.

Soul Searching

I have found that if I shift my inner world, my external world shifts. I think of it as leadership … from the inside.
Michael Rennie

The day before we flew back to Sydney, I went to the markets to say my farewells. In typical Serbian fashion, the stone fruit woman gave me a hug and three kisses: one cheek, then the other cheek, then the first cheek again. It reminded me of crossing the road: look to your right, then to your left, then to your right again.

"Do you like where you live?" she asked.

"Yes."

"Do you *love* where you live?"

"Yes."

"Good. That's very important. I love where I live. We've been through a lot, but that's what teaches you the important things. I have friends who went to live in Australia but they came back after two years. They said Australia didn't have a soul. They said everything looked good but somehow something was missing. A sense of hollowness was in everything—even their fruit and vegetables. They were blemish-free and picture-perfect but they'd lost their flavour. People could buy anything they wanted, but it didn't feel like enough. That's what my friends said, anyway. If you love living there, you must have discovered the soul of the place. Everything and everyone has a soul, if you dig deep enough. Bring your father back again next year," she instructed.

"I will," I promised. As I turned to go she called me back.

"Do you have a man with a good soul?"

"Yes …" I hesitated. "But it's not *his* soul that's the problem."

333

Packing: Take 4

Men for the sake of getting a living forget to live.
Margaret Fuller

I had one last pampering session at the gym on the eve of our return. I exchanged warm farewells with my personal trainers and brow wipers, and walked back home through the hot, dusty streets. It was 11 pm. The gym also kept my kind of hours.

Two blocks from Milica's house, I found myself in total darkness—no street lights and no house lights. I suspected another power failure. I stumbled home over uprooted concrete and fumbled my way through the gate and the front door, and then optimistically flicked a light switch. Nothing. I bumped my way to the living room and found it deserted. Milica was at a christening, while Dad had stayed home to watch a movie. I called out to him, but no-one answered.

The darkness felt as though a black cat had wrapped itself around my head. I couldn't even see my own hand in front of me. I remembered there was a candelabrum above the sofa in the lounge room, and several contusions later I carried it into the kitchen. Luckily, I found matches that the last cigarette-smoking visitor had left on the table. In relief I sank into a chair that wasn't there and fell to the floor. One of the candles broke off the candelabrum, rolled across the floor and dropped down the stairs. I had two candles left. I struck a match and the cat in front of my eyes vanished. I lit the candles, gingerly picked myself up and crept down the stairs. I called out to Dad again—this time he answered.

"What's going on?" I asked. "What are you doing?"

"I've been waiting for you," he replied. "When I finished watching TV, I came downstairs to get ready for bed and suddenly all the lights went out. I couldn't see a thing, so I just sat here and prayed you'd make it home safely."

"I had no idea there was a power failure. Everything was fine at the gym. You must've been sitting here for almost an hour."

"The important thing is that you're home. I guess there's nothing to do but go to bed and hope Milica is OK."

"Actually, we have to pack our bags for tomorrow morning. You hold the candelabrum and light my path, so I can find your things."

With my father dripping hot wax down my neck and arms, we spent an hour rummaging around the room for odd socks and crumpled T-shirts. We then repeated the process in my room. We finished at 1.30 am, just as we heard Milica arrive.

"The construction workers severed the power lines," she reported, as she handed us a dozen candles.

"We noticed," I said.

The power came back on just as we got ourselves to bed.

Whisper

*To forgive is to set a prisoner free and discover
that the prisoner was you.*
Lewis B. Smedes

Give me Belgrade airport any day. Security was all smiles. Our three full water bottles went unnoticed. Why are you taking out a plastic bag containing your toothpaste and contact lens solution? Why are you taking off your shoes? Why are you taking your laptop out of its bag? Unattended luggage littered the departure lounge, and the public address announcements were completely incomprehensible, no matter what language you spoke.

Five minutes before walking through Customs, I remembered that we hadn't returned to the Ministry for Internal Affairs to inform our slow-motion friends of our departure. Milica was unconcerned.

"Give me your ID cards and I'll take them back this afternoon. You'll soon be out of their reach in Australia."

During the first leg of our return journey, from Belgrade to Frankfurt, we managed to work our way through a quarter of the food that Milica had packed. Apparently airline food wouldn't keep a sparrow from starving. Then, during the flight from Frankfurt to Hong Kong, drowsiness overcame me and I even let lapse our life-saving foot flexion exercises.

"Are you awake?" Dad whispered.

I was too tired to respond.

"I love you," he murmured, almost inaudibly.

My eyes shot open. I had not heard this from him in more than
30 years.

Select Bibliography and Recommended Reading

Albom, Mitch. *Tuesdays With Morrie: An old man, a young man, and life's greatest lesson.* Broadway Books, 2002.

Cowan, Graeme. *Back From the Brink Too: Helping your loved one overcome depression.* Bird In Hand Media, 2009.

Doidge MD, Norman. *The Brain That Changes Itself: Stories of personal triumph from the frontiers of brain science.* Scribe Publications, 2010.

Doidge MD, Norman. *The Brain's Way of Healing: Remarkable discoveries and recoveries from the frontiers of neuroplasticity.* Scribe Publications, 2015.

Emmons, Robert. *Thanks! How practising gratitude can make you happier.* Mariner Books, 2008.

Frederickson Ph.D, Barbara L. *Positivity: Top-notch research reveals the 3-to-1 ratio that will change your life.* Three Rivers Press, 2009.

Gladwell, Malcolm. *Blink: The power of thinking without thinking.* Back Bay Books, 2007.

Leunig, Michael. *Poems 1972–2002.* Viking, 2003.

McKissock, Mal & Dianne. *Coping With Grief.* ABC Books, 1995.

Medina, John. *Brain Rules: 12 principles for surviving and thriving at work, home and school.* Pear Press, 2008.

Michie, David. *Hurry Up and Meditate: Your starter kit for inner peace and better health*. Snow Lion Publications, 2008.

Popovic MBBS, Helena. *NeuroSlimming: Let your brain change your body*. Choose Health, 2015

Ratey, Dr John J, & Hagerman, E. *Spark! How exercise will improve the performance of your brain*. Quercus Publishing Plc, 2009.

Rock, David. *Your Brain at Work: Strategies for overcoming distraction, regaining focus and working smarter all day long*. Harper Collins, 2009

Strauch, Barbara. *Secrets of the Grown-Up Brain: The surprising talents of the middle-aged mind*. Black Inc., 2010.

Tolle, Eckhart. *A New Earth: Awakening to your life's purpose*. Penguin, 2005.

Tolle, Eckhart. *Stillness Speaks: A book designed for meditative reading*. New World Library, 2003.

Tolle, Eckhart. *The Power of Now: A guide to spiritual enlightenment*. New World Library, 2004.

Valenzuela, Dr Michael J. *It's Never Too Late to Change Your Mind: The latest medical thinking on what you can do to avoid dementia*. ABC Books, 2009.

Wiles & Wiles, Judith & Janet. *The Memory Book: Everyday habits for a healthy memory*. ABC Books, 2003.

Useful Websites

adventurepreventsdementia.com

winningatslimming.com

drhelenapopovic.com

dementia.org.au

dementiacareinternational.com

brainhq.com

carersaustralia.com.au

mensshed.org